Skinny Without Willpower

Skinny Without Willpower

Yogesh Verma

Yogesh Verma
630 Palomino Dr., Pleasanton, CA 94566
yogeshv@hotmail.com, Phone: 510 364-5177

www.SkinnyWithoutWillpower.com

Editor Sally Wolfe
Copyeditor Mary Harris
Formatted by Tamara Cribley
Cover Design by Fiona Jayde
Illustrations by Samantha Lai and Tanisha Verma
Author Photograph by Rajesh Verma

ISBN: 978-0-9973794-0-2

DISCLAIMER

The information contained in this book is solely for informational and educational purposes, and any advice should be taken as such. The suggestions presented are not meant to cure any medical condition or ailment. All health matters should be supervised by a personal physician or a qualified health practitioner who is familiar with your health status. Please consult your physician before changing any diet or exercise regimen because only your physician can provide you with medical advice. Yogesh Verma disclaims any liability or warranties of any kind arising directly or indirectly from the use of the information contained in this book.

Any mention of specific companies, organizations, or authorities in the book doesn't imply endorsement by the author or the publisher or vice versa.

Praise for Yogesh

I used to have high lipids and was busy taking statins to manage it. I took them for a couple of years, and while my lipids got in control, my fasting sugar started to climb. For a while I tried following the "prescribed" diet of low-cholesterol, low-fat and low-sugar, along with few different drugs but didn't make much progress. Even some exercise could not change much. I finally decided to take things in my control and on Yogesh's suggestions; I neglected the low-fat, low-cholesterol diet for a while, and against my doctor's will, I even stopped my statin prescription. Substituted low fat/cholesterol breakfasts with eggs, nuts, cheese, butter, and whole milk. Followed it for few months—and along with some exercise—I was able to bring down my total cholesterol from 255 to <210. I then started monitoring my post-meal blood sugar. I experimented with lot of different food types and portions. The whole concept of glycemic index is definitely quite reliable. I could eat 4 eggs or a large portion of Chicken Caesar salad for lunch and my blood-sugar would hardly change. But just a can of cola would make it touch 200. Since last 2 months I have been watching my diet and limiting simple carbs and my fasting blood sugar has dropped from >116 to <102. I feel energetic all throughout the day and feel good to get in control without the use of synthetic chemicals. Good I listened to Yogesh and tried his AXIOM suggestions. I still have some ways to go but I'm definitely on the right path.

RV, San Ramon CA

Yogesh! Thanks a ton for getting me started on this path... I know I am just a beginner...but I finally see some hope. For those of you who don't know me... I am a 44-year-old woman struggling to stay fit for more than half my life. I have been suffering from "Fibromyalgia" for more than two years and almost gave up on exercising...To top that, I have been diagnosed with Sleep Apnea... and have major sleep issues! Am always exhausted—and in pain, a state that I refuse to be in because I have a fulltime job and a little one to take care of! I started on this diet I call "Yogi's diet" ... about six weeks ago. Being a vegetarian, I wondered what the hell I will eat without rice or wheat. But with Yogesh's guidance, I have been easily able to call off carbs for all this duration. No temptations what so ever! I am enjoying eating the foods I avoided before like Ghee, nuts, coconut, paneer; I actually found that I have more choices now. My energy level has really picked up. I am able to exercise. I lost about 7 pounds. I am finally seeing some light at the end of the tunnel and am very optimistic that I am headed in the right direction! I appreciate all your time and patience, Yogesh! You are always available to answer any silly question I have! THANK YOU!

HG, New York, NY

After trying out several different diets, I realized I was not getting very far. They would work for a while and then the weight would come right back. One day, I found myself listening to my dear friend Yogesh's advice about how to customize and stick to a diet and make it work for you in the long term. He explained to me how diets work and suggested methods that helped me formulate a weight loss diet.

I am now following all of his tips about losing weight. Within 2 months, I have lost 27 pounds. Yogesh's diet also helped me maintain my weight. I am looking forward to the release of his forthcoming book *Skinny Without Willpower*.

MS, Livermore, CA

Yogesh has been very influential in my journey to a flat belly. I'd like to share a few quick things, based on his direction and coaching, that helped me achieve the goal. Though there is more to do, I am quite happy with the results so far...

Drastically reduce sugars and processed foods. Follow a Low Carb High Fat pattern. Lots of veggies. Following his pyramid for Carbs/Fats & Protein...This resulted in belly shrinking from 34 (pants waist size) to 32 and then 30. Then came a trip to India and size was back to about 33 but now is back to 30. So I know that we can fall off the wagon but can quickly get back on it.

A ton of gratitude to Yogesh for showing the path that worked for me. His immense knowledge in nutrition and his willingness to share it for greater good is quite commendable. Thank you Yogesh!!!

EY, Sacramento, CA

I have been on Yogesh's diet for the past 3 weeks and my motivation was to lose the belly fat I gained due to stress. In three weeks, I have lost 3 kg and most of my belly fat. The best part I like about his diet is that I can eat many of my favorite foods and I don't have to count calories or serving size. I enjoy the foods and don't worry about cutting calories and I lose weight at the same time. My energy levels are high and I even get to cheat on my favorite desserts and indulgence foods every now and then.

Thank you, Yogesh, for helping me lose the stubborn belly fat. You are indeed very approachable, friendly, and supportive at any point of time. You proved that distance is not the constraint in reaching out to people and help to achieve the goal.

Thank you once again.

VM, Bangalore, India

Thank you for helping me lose 3kgs in not more than 12-20 days. And not to forget the stubborn belly fat that was also lost.

SA, New Delhi, India

Dedicated to my parents, who taught me that anything was possible if I believed in myself. Thank you, Mummy and Dada, for encouraging me and supporting me unconditionally through the twists and turns of life and thank you for believing in me more than I did in myself.

Table of Contents

Appendixes: Reference Material

Acknowledgements

This book is the culmination of fifteen years of scouring nutrition research and experimenting with diet and lifestyle changes in my and several others' lives, and understanding the health outcomes of these changes. During these years, several people have been key in inspiring me to write this book. This a small attempt at thanking those people in no particular order of importance.

My first manuscript was over 300 pages, with over 250 references that looked more like a research dissertation than a book. It covered nutrition for most chronic ailments such as diabetes, heart disease, age-related dementia, and cancer. When I first sent the manuscript to my editor Sally Wolfe, she encouraged me to focus on one subject so that it appealed to a particular reader. "Write a book that solves one problem that people face," she said. That's when I began rewriting my book in its current form to focus on one of the biggest myths that surrounds weight loss: *"eat less and exercise more."* Sally was patient with me and slowly (but painfully for her) turned me from a technical writer to a writer who the common person could understand. Thank you, Sally, for giving me a voice people can understand.

My special thanks to my dear friends Devalok Girdhar and Arvind Girdhar for introducing me to carbohydrate conscious eating several years ago. Once I started blogging, I was encouraged by several friends to put all the information in the form of a book. Most notable among them were, Sujatha Kattimani, Suresh Palliparambil Menon, and Balaji Girisiballa. Also, my special thanks to Subraya Mallya for designing my blog inutrifit.com.

My special thanks to my cover designer Fiona Jayde (fionajaydemedia.com) for designing the cute, catchy cover. Also thanks to Mary Harris (maryharriswriter.com) who patiently copyedited my work and taught me the legalities of copyrights. Thanks to Tamara Cribley (deliberatepage.com) for formatting the book to various formats. Thanks to Samantha Lai and my daughter, Tanisha Verma, for the illustrations. Thanks to my brother Rajesh Verma for the author picture. Thanks to my son Shashwat Verma for the social media management for this book.

It goes without saying that I couldn't have written this book without learning myself from the writings of eminent authors before me. This work stands on the shoulders of greats like Dr. David Ludwig (*Always Hungry?*), Dr. Robert Lustig (*Fat Chance*), Gary Taubes (*Good Calories, Bad Calories* and *Why We Get Fat*), Dr. Malcolm Kendrick (*The Great Cholesterol Con*), Dr. Uffe Ravnskov (*Ignore the Awkward*), Dr. William Davis (*Wheat Belly*) and Mark Sisson (*The Primal Blueprint*).

Furthermore, my special thanks to eminent researchers in the field of human nutrition, Dr. Christopher Gardner (Director of Nutrition Studies at Stanford Prevention Research Center and Professor of Medicine at Stanford University), Dr. Robert Lustig (Professor at UCSF School of Medicine), and Dr. David Ludwig (Professor of Nutrition at Harvard School of Public Health) for patiently answering my questions on hormonal interactions of diet.

Not to mention that without the support of my family this work couldn't have been complete so I thank my wife Anuja and kids Shashwat and Tanisha for understanding the many evenings and weekends that I spent writing, away from them. So thank you for understanding me and bearing with me.

Thanks to my brother Rajesh Verma, my brother-in-law Lokesh Verma and to my good friends, Himabindu Gurla, Eman Yarlagadda, Murugavel Sambandhan, Balaji Girisaballa, and several others for being the early adopters of my diet and believing in my dietary suggestions even though it flew in the face of conventional wisdom. Their positive results and encouragement kept me motivated to continue writing. And lastly I owe a special thanks to all the people worldwide that trust in my advice and follow my dietary suggestions to stay healthy. Without the positive reinforcement from all of you this book wouldn't have been possible.

Thanks to all of you! Stay happy, healthy and prosperous!

Prologue

"If you tell a lie big enough and keep repeating it, people will eventually come to believe it..."

Joseph Goebbels

How many times have you heard that *"eating fat will make you fat,"* or, in order to lose weight you have to *"eat less and exercise more"*? More times than you can remember, right? For nearly forty years, we have been told that in order to lose weight, we have to avoid fat and cut calories while at the same time increase the amount of activity or exercise. Weight loss, according to the experts, is nothing more than a math problem of calories in (food intake) minus calories out (activity or exercise). Any excess or deficit between the two shows up as an increase or decrease in body weight! Fat, having more than twice the number of calories, gram for gram, compared to carbohydrate or protein, makes a prime candidate to eliminate in one's diet, in order to cut excess calories.

In accordance with this advice, we have been cutting fat from our diets by eating fat-free factory foods that your great-grandma wouldn't recognize. At the same time, we have been spending endless hours on the treadmill. We have become a calorie-counting society, and almost every American adult has some calorie-counting app on his or her smartphone and you can't drive a block without finding a fitness club or a gym. Yet, our waistlines continue to expand and we continue to push the scales.

This trend is aptly represented in the chart below from Centers for Disease Control and Prevention (CDC) that shows the US obesity trend from 1960 until 2004.

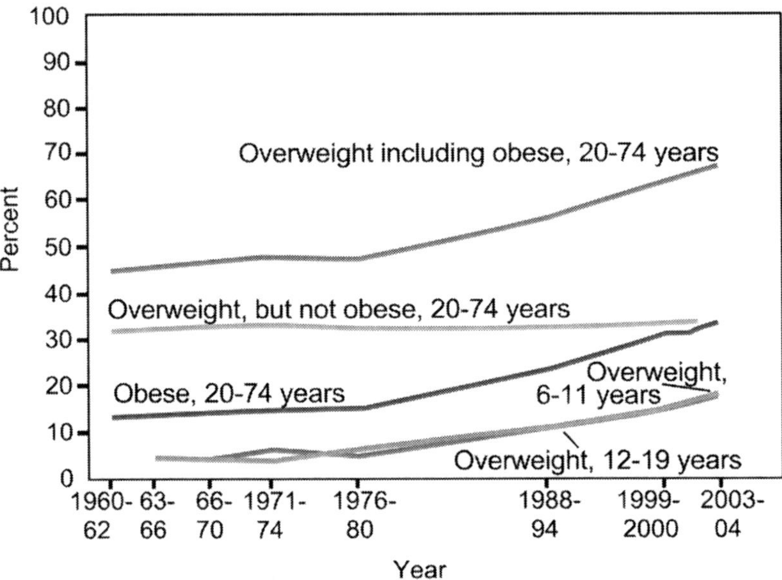

Figure 1: Overweight and obese, by age: United States, 1960–1962 through 2003–2004 (Source: Centers for Disease Control and Prevention, National Center for Health Statistics, Health, United States, 2006, Figure 13, Data from National Health and Nutrition Examination Survey).

According to the US Department of Health and Human Services, 2 out of 3 adults are overweight, 1 in 3 adults are obese and about one-third of the children and adolescents between the ages of 6-19 are overweight or obese. Obviously, something is not working in spite of us following the expert advice.

One thing that is pretty clear from Figure 1: right around 1980, the obesity rates across all age groups shot up. Is it just a matter of coincidence that right around that time the US Department of Agriculture (USDA) put out the nutritional guidelines that advised all Americans to cut the amount of dietary fat and instead get more calories from starches and grains in the form of rice, pasta, potatoes, cereals, and crackers? This later on took the form of the famous USDA Pyramid, shown in Figure 2, which put fat on top of the pyramid in the "*eat sparingly*" category while carbohydrate got a seat in the bottom of the pyramid in the "*eat plentiful*" category.

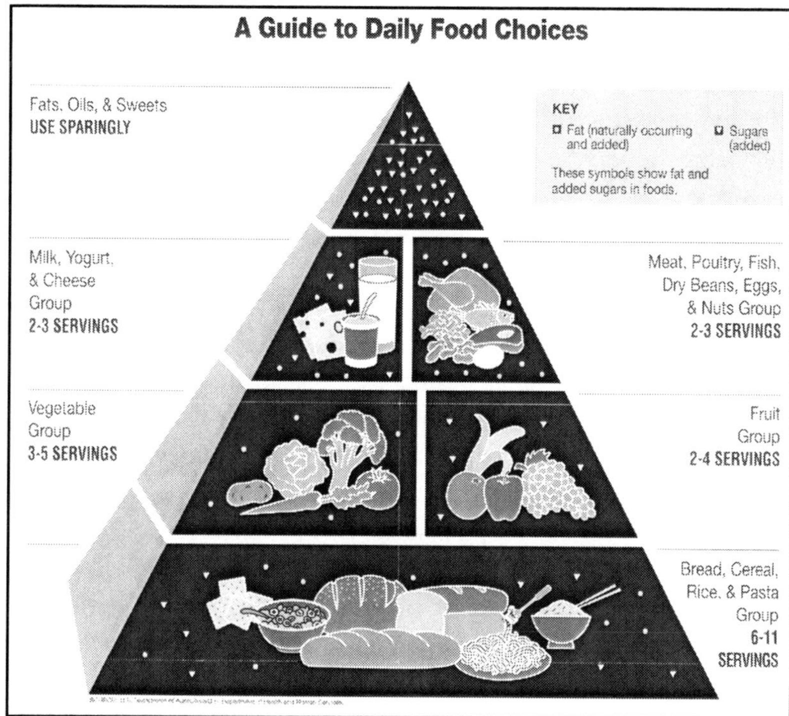

Figure 2: USDA Food Pyramid (Source: US Department of Agriculture/US Department of Health and Human Services.

This makes one wonder if the advice given to us by the USDA was right in the first place. As you shall see in this book, this nutritional advice led to the fattening of America and the rest of the world. Along with this came the wave of obesity-related diseases like diabetes, heart disease, blood pressure, osteoarthritis, fatty liver disease, sleep apnea, and the list goes on and on.

The simplistic advice of "*eating less and exercising more*" makes a lot of sense on the surface. After all, if you burn more calories than you eat, you should lose weight, right? It's the first law of thermodynamics, plain and simple!

As you read through the book, you will realize why this apparently simple math doesn't work in the human body and why nature doesn't allow it in the long run.

The book is divided into two parts. In Part 1, you will learn about the real underlying causes of weight gain. You will learn how the current Western processed diet has contributed to the rise in obesity, how it has shifted our bodies into fat storage mode, and why our bodies won't respond to our earnest efforts at losing weight. You will also see why losing weight is not simply a matter of "willpower," and that no amount of "willpower" will get you to lose weight unless you alter the composition of your diet. You will learn how our current diet has altered our hormonal profile to favor weight gain. We are essentially prisoners of our hormones, and this book will show you how to break free from your hormonal prison and lose weight effortlessly.

In Part 2, you will learn simple practical tips that you can implement in your diet and lifestyle in order to lose weight effortlessly. No more calorie counting and no more spending endless hours at the gym.

The Appendices have useful information like belly fat busting superfoods, glycemic index and antioxidant content of common foods, high quality protein sources for vegetarians and a lot of other useful information for the serious reader: on dietary fat and cholesterol, and chronic disease prevention that goes beyond weight loss.

Weight loss doesn't have to be torturous deprivation and endless sweating. Weight loss can be effortless and enjoyable. In this book, I want to show you how you can unlock your own fat-burning potential and transform yourself into a leaner, healthier you. You CAN be *Skinny Without Willpower!*

Yogesh Verma, PhD, CNT
Pleasanton, California
February, 2016

Introduction

When Heather first called me, she was going through a painful divorce. She was stressed most of the time, and to make matters worse, she was suffering from fibromyalgia and sleep apnea. She was 44 years old and had struggled to stay fit half her life. She was always tired and in pain. As a result, exercising was almost impossible. She was on pain meds just to stay functional. Desperate to lose weight, she cut calories, but her weight didn't budge. Nothing seemed to help.

When we talked, she didn't sound too hopeful, but was willing to try my suggestions. She figured there wasn't much to lose.

I devised a nutrition plan for her so she could enjoy her favorite foods and not be in a constant state of deprivation. She seemed excited since she could eat her favorite foods with the exception of a few healthy substitutions, such as yams instead of potatoes, quinoa instead of rice, and barley bread instead of wheat bread. I didn't recommend any exercise, but she said she was going to use the stationary bike.

Two weeks later, I heard back.

"I lost three pounds and I feel great," she chirped.

She was still on pain meds but was optimistic that if her progress continued, she could attempt to reduce the dosage. I recommended some herbal anti-inflammatory supplements to lessen her pain.

Three weeks passed, and I got another call from her.

"I have lost another four pounds!"

"How's your pain?" I asked her.

"My pain has subsided enough for me to cut my meds in half. Also my energy levels are up and I'm using the bike every day."

"That's great!" I said.

She said she hadn't felt this good in years and added she was getting compliments on how radiant she was looking.

When I first spoke to Roger about his health issues, weight gain was only one of them. What worried him more was his high cholesterol and fasting blood sugar levels. He had a family history of diabetes and heart disease, so it was a serious concern. He had followed a low-fat/low-cholesterol diet, but it wasn't lowering his cholesterol or his weight. He was on cholesterol meds and his fasting sugar levels were edging higher. Exercise didn't seem to have any effect. I asked him to abandon the low-fat/low-cholesterol diet and recommended a diet of wholesome natural fats and healthy proteins. Exercise was optional.

A few months later, he reported that he was completely off medications and his cholesterol had dropped from over 255 to less than 210. During the same time, his fasting blood sugar levels also dropped from over 116 to 102. The best part, he said, was that he was able to enjoy his favorite foods (eggs, butter, cheese, whole milk) and felt completely in control of his health.

Heather and Roger suffered from different symptoms, but weight gain was a common problem for both. Following the dietary prescriptions, they both lost weight and got rid of their "other" symptoms as well. It's essential not to treat weight gain as an isolated problem. The goal was wellness; weight loss was a pleasant side effect.

This is the book for you if you are:

- Overweight and have struggled unsuccessfully to lose weight.
- Crave sweet, salty, and fried foods.
- Depressed, exhausted, and sick most of the time.
- Suffering from high cholesterol and blood sugar.
- Ready to thrive!

What makes people fat?

Let me start out by asking you this question:

What do you believe makes people fat?

a) Laziness
b) Overeating
c) Eating fat
d) All of the above
e) None of the above

Almost everyone I ask this question of responds with **d) all of the above**.

We have been told by the experts that weight gain is a consequence of the double sin of gluttony and lethargy. Whenever we see an overweight person, we automatically assume that they must be lazy and must be overeating.

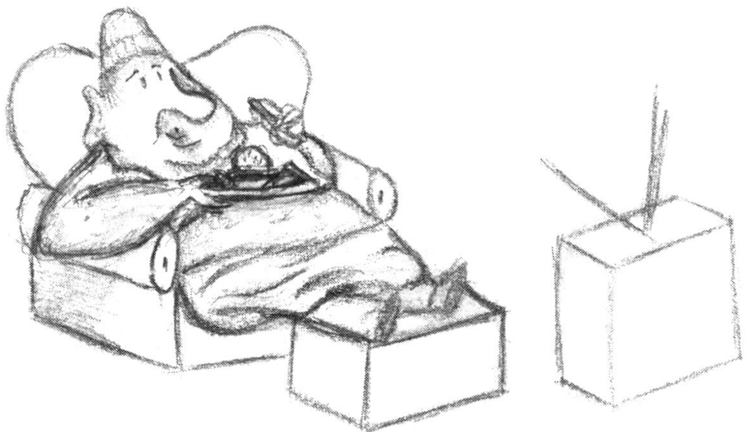

Figure 3: The double sin of gluttony and lethargy is blamed as the main reason for obesity

Contrary to popular notion, the surprising answer—and the answer that led me to write this book—is **e**).

Weight gain is neither a result of overeating nor a result of laziness, and the purpose of this book is to demonstrate why.

My hope is that my own search and discovery of this truth will help you achieve your ideal weight and unlock your true health potential.

You Too Can Do It: My Story

I was overweight and identified with high cholesterol at the age of 26. My doctor advised me to start taking cholesterol-lowering medication, go on a low-fat diet, and reduce calories.

I declined the medication and decided to focus on lifestyle changes. I started exercising. I shunned fat and embraced everything non-fat in the hope of losing weight and lowering my cholesterol. I followed the United States Department of Agriculture (USDA) food pyramid (Figure 2) to the letter, eating mostly bread, cereals, rice, wheat, and pasta while avoiding fat and animal products like the plague.

The weight kept piling on. In four years, I went from 176 to 220 pounds! My cholesterol hit 250! Blood tests revealed high fasting sugar levels and high triglycerides. I also suffered from early-morning ankle pains. Everything about my health pointed me toward a life of diabetes and heart disease and who knows what else. My maternal grandfather was diabetic and a heart patient and died at the age of 56 from a massive heart attack, so I knew I had the genes for it.

When my first child was born, I decided to make another change.

I decided to do my own research.

I embarked on a serious campaign of study. I devoured the scientific literature: on fats, carbohydrates, proteins, and basic human biochemistry. Researching something is like peeling an onion. You keep peeling layers and layers and it seems the deeper you go, the juicier it gets. The more I read, the more I realized that the advice given today by the medical community has little to do with the actual science of nutrition and more to do with the commerce and politics of food!

What I discovered: The truths about weight gain and about fat and cholesterol are buried deep beneath the food politics and popular press that has glorified low-fat dogma and maligned the real facts for years.

What I Learned

Contrary to the doctor-recommended USDA diet, fat and cholesterol are actually vital to health. But other people's research wasn't enough for me. I experimented; I wanted to find out for myself.

In the beginning, I started replacing some of the calories from bread, rice, and pasta with healthy fats from nuts, avocados, and olive oil. I even started eating butter and ghee (clarified butter) in moderation. I wasn't actually "dieting" (cutting calories) but replacing carbohydrates with healthy fats. I also upped my protein intake from fish and organic free-pastured poultry and meats, further replacing some of the carbohydrate calories.

So instead of eating according to the USDA food pyramid (recommended 50% carb, 30% fat, and 20% protein calories[1]), I was eating about equal proportions of fat, protein, and carbohydrate.

Dramatic changes occurred. My moods got better, and I was full of energy. I stopped having hunger pangs between meals, and my weight started to come down. So did my cholesterol, fasting blood sugar, and triglycerides. Even my skin was more radiant (or so I was told). The early morning ankle pains also disappeared.

I was rejuvenated!

Ever since then, I have helped dozens of people lose weight and realize a higher state of health. I started blogging at inutrifit.com and pretty soon, I was helping numerous people all around the world with dietary advice to combat weight issues and chronic disease.

At the urging of my close friends and family, I decided to write this book. My goal is to show you how you can lose weight without going on a restrictive diet and enjoy the foods you like. And even beyond that, my goal is to help you realize a higher state of wellbeing. In one word, I want you to "thrive."

PART 1

UNDERSTANDING THE CAUSES

CHAPTER 1

Willpower vs. The Mighty Calorie: Why Weight Loss Diets Fail

"The concept of the "calorie," as applied to nutrition is an oversimplification so extreme as to be untrue in practice."

J. Stanton, *The Gnoll Credo*

In this chapter, you will learn:

- Why reducing calories is disastrous to weight loss
- Why exercising more doesn't work either

We are all familiar with the mighty calorie: the No #1 enemy of anyone trying to lose weight. The familiar axiom is to eat as few calories as possible and burn as many as possible. It's as if the moment these little buggers enter our bodies, they go and hide in all the unsightly places where fat exists.

CALORIES
Sneaky tiny creatures that live in
your closet and sew your clothes
a little bit tighter every night

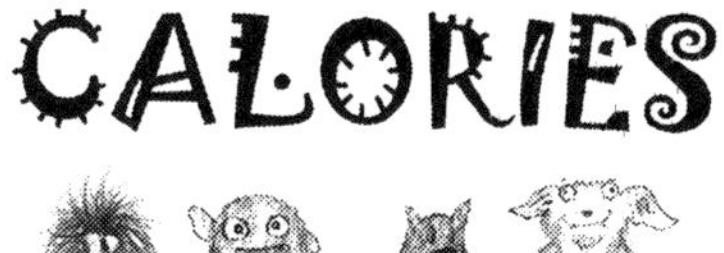

Figure 4: The dreaded mighty calorie

Let's take a closer look at the mighty calorie and see why we fear it so much.

A calorie is nothing but a unit of energy that we need for survival. The food we eat provides us with energy to sustain vital functions (breathing, thinking, heart beating, digesting, etc.). It also provides us with energy to work. The problem occurs when there are excess calories left over from food that aren't used. These excess calories convert to stored body fat.

> Hunger and metabolism are always striving to achieve your weight set-point via *homeostasis.*

The problem is that we think of weight loss as a math problem. Cut the amount of calories and your body will have to turn to its own reserves of stored body fat to fill the energy deficit. Calories consumed minus the calories burnt equals weight loss (or gain). This is called the calorie in/calorie out (CICO) hypothesis of weight loss. Hence, we hear the familiar weight loss advice:

"Eat less and exercise more."

Let's look closer why this simplistic model of weight loss doesn't add up.

Your Weight Set-Point and Homeostasis

The human body doesn't behave like a black box of calories in which you take out more than you put in and weight loss results. This is due to a phenomenon called *homeostasis*, or equilibrium. All life on this planet operates on the principle of *homeostasis*. For example, the body maintains a certain internal temperature. When the external environment gets too hot, the body cools down by sweating (evaporation of sweat causes cooling). When it gets too cold outside, the body generates heat by shivering. Same goes for the pH of blood, which is maintained at a set value. Simply put, nature always strives to achieve a set-point by balancing two opposing forces (heat and cold, acidity and alkalinity). Sort of like being in a tug of war with equals. If one force pulls harder on one side, the other force pulls equally harder such that balance is maintained.

The same goes for your energy (or calorie) needs that are regulated by the forces of hunger and metabolism. Hunger is the force that puts energy (calories) into your body and metabolism (or activity level) is the force that consumes or takes away energy (calories) from your body. Hunger and metabolism are always striving to achieve your weight set-point via ***homeostasis***. Think of these two forces as the yin and yang of weight loss.

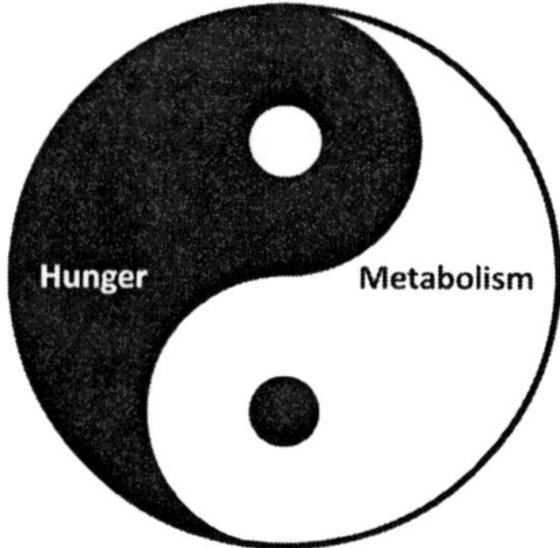

Figure 5: The opposing forces of hunger and metabolism to maintain homeostasis

This brings us to two of the greatest myths of weight loss.

Myth 1: Eat Less to Lose Weight

When you eat less than what your body requires, it sends powerful signals to the brain to ramp up hunger to fulfill the body's energy needs. When you exert willpower and ignore the hunger signals, the brain counteracts by suppressing your basal metabolism[A] so that you burn fewer calories. You essentially go into calorie-saving mode. In order to suppress basal metabolism (activity level), the brain sacrifices muscle tissue that provides the immediate energy needs via stored glycogen (a form of glucose that is stored in the muscle tissue for a quick source of energy), in the absence of food.

This is why you lose muscle before you lose fat when you go on an "eat less" diet. Losing muscle drops your metabolism and makes you lazy. The end result is you become hungry and listless.

Bottom line is, if you exert "willpower" to defeat your hunger, you end up sacrificing metabolism by losing muscle tissue. Without glycogen in the muscles, you are incapable of any activity, which leads to lethargy.

A The basal metabolism is the amount of energy required by your vital organs to function: heart (to pump blood), brain (to think), liver (to process various macronutrients), stomach (to digest food), and your muscles (to move).

Since you lose muscle before you lose fat, and since muscle is denser than fat, the initial weight loss is rapid. But losing weight by losing muscle is not sustainable in the long run. If your calorie needs aren't met, you keep cannibalizing muscle and your metabolism keeps dropping. So the more you exert willpower and forgo eating the slower your metabolism gets and the lazier you become. Soon you have no energy to do anything and life's demands and your own flailing willpower catch up to you and you succumb to your natural eating habits. Then the weight comes back as fast as it left. But here is a twist. When you eat less, the primal brain instincts assume you are in a famine situation. The body wants to protect itself from such famine situation, so it prefers to gain fat over muscle. Hence, you gain more fat and some of the muscle you initially lost. Remember, nature doesn't care for your health; all it cares about is your survival. And having stored body fat is the best survival tool in a famine.

Essentially, eating less makes you fat in the long run!

This is the beginning of the weight loss tragedy set in motion by the simplistic assumption of eating less to lose weight.

The next time you go on a "eat less" diet, the amount of muscle to cannibalize is less than the first time. So the weight loss isn't as dramatic. Each time you diet, you lose more muscle, and when you break the diet, you gain more fat. Slowly your body fat percentage goes up, and losing weight with each round becomes harder.

Reality 1

Studies show that you gain an average of 11 pounds for every diet you go on. Essentially, eating less makes you fat in the long run!

Myth 2: Exercise More to Lose Weight

This is the flip side of Myth 1, as exercise is another way to put your body in a calorie deficit. Just like thirst (after sweating), hunger is ramped up to maintain *homeostasis* after exercise-related calorie loss. So you get hungry after a vigorous bout of exercise. If you were to go by natural instincts, you would eat accordingly and regain the lost calories and no net weight loss would happen. The more vigorous the exercise, the more voracious the appetite it induces. Most people who lose weight from exercising do so because once again, they exert "*willpower*" and stop themselves from eating lost calories. Plus, they make judicious choices in food; for example, skipping the donut and eating a salad. So exercise by itself cannot cause weight loss unless it's backed up with willpower to eat less. More on this subject in Chapter 5.

Reality 2

Eating less and exercising more are mutually exclusive, meaning if you eat less, you cannot exercise more and vice versa. So "eat less and exercise more" is really an oxymoron.

Willpower is Finite

The reason why most people are unsuccessful at losing weight by eating less and exercising more is because the amount of "willpower" is finite. Nature never gets tired in its pursuit of homeostasis, but "willpower" eventually crumbles. We eventually give up and succumb to hunger and regain the lost weight. It may take you weeks or months or even years, but eventually most of us will get back to our "natural" weight.

To summarize, we can't lose weight just by consuming fewer calories than we need because of the opposing forces of HUNGER and METABOLISM.

Sounds pretty abysmal, doesn't it? Don't lose hope, because there is a way out and that's what I want to show you.

CHAPTER 2

Why We Get Fat: Carbohydrate Metabolism

"There is nothing more deceptive than an obvious fact."

Arthur Conan Doyle

In this chapter, you will learn:

- The real reason behind weight gain.
- Why eating fat by itself cannot make you fat.
- How certain foods are responsible for driving up hunger and causing weight gain.
- How those same foods are also highly addictive.

Let's examine the real reason why we gain weight. First, you need to understand how your body metabolizes energy and stores fat. It will revolutionize your thinking and your life.

Our diet has three major components: carbohydrates, fat, and protein. **Carbohydrates** mainly serve the purpose of fuel, because they are nothing but large chains of sugar molecules. **Proteins** (and amino acids) are the building blocks of all cells and tissues. **Fats** are the basic building blocks of hormones and form an integral part of all cell membranes. Additionally fats help transport the fat-soluble vitamins A, D, E, and K witch serve several vital functions in our body.

How these three components work together is the story of metabolism and weight regulation. One of the main characters of this story is a hormone called insulin. Essentially, the role of insulin is that of sugar police, whose job it is to keep excess sugar out of your blood circulation. When you eat more carbohydrates than your body can use, you set off the insulin alarm—and the carbohydrates that you don't use are turned into stored body fat! So the important question is, as you're probably thinking, how do I stop the alarm from going off?

Let's take a look at how all this works.

Understanding Carbohydrates: How Sugar Becomes Fat

Insulin regulates the sugar in our body. Carbohydrates play a vital role in controlling how much sugar is in the blood at any given time by stimulating the production of insulin in the pancreas. When we eat food, the carbohydrates get broken down into sugar molecules in the gut and get absorbed in the bloodstream as blood glucose. A normal healthy adult has about 5 grams (a teaspoon) of sugar in 5 liters of blood (the average volume of blood in an adult). This translates to 100 mg/dl[B] of blood sugar, which is the threshold of fasting blood sugar for a non-diabetic person. Fasting blood sugar is the amount of glucose in your blood after 8 to 12 hours of not eating.

Whenever the amount of total sugar in the blood goes above a teaspoon, the pancreas secretes insulin. The liver, on insulin's command, converts this excess sugar into glycogen and stores some of it for later use to fuel the brain in the absence of food, say, when you are sleeping. In the absence of carbohydrates, the liver can metabolize fats and proteins to generate glucose for the purpose of energy. The remaining glycogen is sent to muscle tissue to be stored for immediate energy needs. Any leftover glycogen is then converted in the liver (again on insulin's command) to tiny droplets of fat (known as triglycerides). These triglyceride molecules are then stored into adipose tissue as body fat.

Insulin: Master Storage Hormone

Insulin is known as the master storage hormone. The only way to activate insulin in your body is by eating carbohydrates (and to some extent protein). To demonstrate this fact, researchers[2] tested the glucose and insulin response to a pure carbohydrate (100g) and a pure fat (40g) meal. In the

B 1 liter has 10 deciliters (dl) and 1 gram has 1000 milligrams (mg).

first group, test subjects were fed a meal of only carbohydrates. The second group ate a meal of only fats. The first group had a quick rise in blood glucose level and a resultant rise in insulin level. In the second group, however, there was no rise in blood glucose level and as a result, no insulin response either! In other words eating fat by itself didn't raise blood glucose levels and as a result the insulin levels didn't rise either. And without insulin there cannot be any weight gain!

Insulin-driven fat storage is the primary mechanism of weight gain.

This proves that fat doesn't make you fat, but carbohydrates do! It's kind of astounding, isn't it?

Fat that we eat is broken down into smaller fatty acids that can be directly used up for energy at the point of use without the need for insulin. So much for the "*eating fat will make you fat*" myth!

The basic fat storage mechanism can be summarized as a three-step process:

1) Carbohydrates in your diet cause an increase in blood sugar levels;
2) Insulin is released in response to excess blood sugar; and
3) Excess unused blood sugar is stored in the fat cells.

So the bottom line is this: Insulin-driven fat storage is the primary mechanism of weight gain. In fact, diabetics with undiagnosed diabetes rapidly lose weight in spite of keeping the same diet mainly because their pancreas is unable to secrete the weight gain hormone insulin.

Chronic Carbohydrate Consumption and Metabolic Syndrome

Early in a person's life, this process of insulin secretion and excess blood sugar storage is very efficient. Eat carbohydrates => blood sugar goes up => insulin is secreted => insulin stores excess blood sugar => sugar level returns to normal => repeat eating carbohydrates, and so on and so forth. What happens when this pattern of eating carbohydrates becomes a habit? Like with everything excessive in the body, slowly the liver, muscle, and fat cells become desensitized to insulin's signals. As years go by, more insulin is needed in order to do the same job of storing excess blood sugar. Just as a habitual coffee drinker needs more and more coffee to produce the same effect as years ago, so do the cells need more and more insulin as time goes on. This is the beginning of insulin resistance.

The irony is that the liver and muscle cells are the first ones to get resistant to insulin's storage commands, which leaves the fat cells to do all the job of storing the excess blood sugar. This is the beginning of obesity.

Furthermore, the fat cells in our midsection, especially in the deeper layers around our vital organs (also known as visceral fat), have a higher number of insulin receptors and are exposed to higher blood circulation. As a result, they have the highest sensitivity to insulin's fat storage command[3]. As insulin resistance spreads to our peripheral fat cells (in our arms and legs), the fat cells in our midsection are busy storing the excess blood sugar. This is a telltale sign of someone with insulin resistance when he or she has excess fat predominantly in the midsection.

Eventually, even the fat cells in the midsection become resistant to insulin's commands, and in that case, the person's blood sugar level stays high even though the whole system is awash with insulin. At this point, both insulin and blood sugar levels are simultaneously high.

This condition is known as Metabolic Syndrome or Syndrome X[4]. According to Stanford professor and eminent diabetes researcher, Dr. Gerald Reaven, the condition is characterized by high insulin and blood sugar levels along with high triglycerides and central (midsection) obesity[5]. This increases your risk for diabetes, coronary heart disease (CHD), and stroke.

Metabolic syndrome shouldn't be confused with type II diabetes, though it is known to be a precursor. Both are characterized by high blood sugar levels, but in type II diabetes, insulin production is completely ceased because the pancreas eventually gives up producing any insulin.

19th Century Cure for Obesity

Ironically, the fact that carbohydrates cause weight gain has been known for almost two centuries. In 1825, Jean Anthelme Brillat-Savarin, French gourmand, described the cure for obesity: "...that a more or less rigid abstinence from everything that is starchy or floury will lead to the lessening of weight."

Brillat-Savarin didn't know anything about insulin at the time, and it wasn't until almost a century later that Fredrick Banting and Charles H. Best discovered insulin[6] and demonstrated its pivotal role in energy storage and regulation. Later, Elliott P. Joslin's pioneering work on *Diabetes Mellitus*[7], first published in 1916, stressed the role of carbohydrates in weight gain, and the initiation and progression of diabetes

Does that mean all carbohydrates are bad and should be eliminated from our diets? Actually, no. Carbohydrates are an important source of many vitamins and antioxidants, especially in fruits and vegetables and should be an integral part of any healthy diet.

Let's take a closer look.

Good Carb, Bad Carb

The quality of a carbohydrate, with respect to its ability to make you gain weight, is determined by how fast it raises blood sugar levels. The sooner your blood sugar level goes up, the sooner insulin-driven fat storage happens. This property is represented by its glycemic index (GI). GI is a relative measure of how fast a given carbohydrate raises your blood sugar compared to pure glucose (assigned an arbitrary GI value of 100).

Potatoes, for example, have a GI of 80, and kick your blood sugar up very fast. Lentils typically have a GI of 30-40, and cause your blood sugar to rise slowly. Fat and meats have a GI of zero since there is no carbohydrate present in them. A GI less than 55 is considered low; a GI of 55-70 is considered moderate; and GI of over 70 is considered high.

GI is not only affected by how much carbohydrate a given serving of food has, but also by the way it's prepared. A boiled potato has a GI of 80, but mashed potato has a GI of 108! GI is also affected by what other ingredients are present in the food along with the carbohydrate (more in the next chapter).

Here's the main point: *The higher the Glycemic Index, the more it promotes fat storage.*

How Carbohydrates Drive up Hunger

The GI value of a carbohydrate has deeper implications about how you gain weight than the simple insulin-driven fat storage mechanism. This can be understood by insulin response time to a given carb. When there is a sudden surge of blood sugar from a high GI carb, the pancreas has to release a lot of insulin (spike) in order to quickly store away the blood sugar. The pancreas essentially goes into panic mode. In the process of doing so, insulin is typically over-produced, so when all the blood sugar is stored away there is leftover insulin in the blood that keeps removing sugar from the blood. This causes the blood sugar to drop below normal baseline levels (the one teaspoon level in an adult) and the person feels lethargic and experiences hunger pangs (shaded area in Figure 6). As a result the person goes for another (typically high GI) carbohydrate meal.

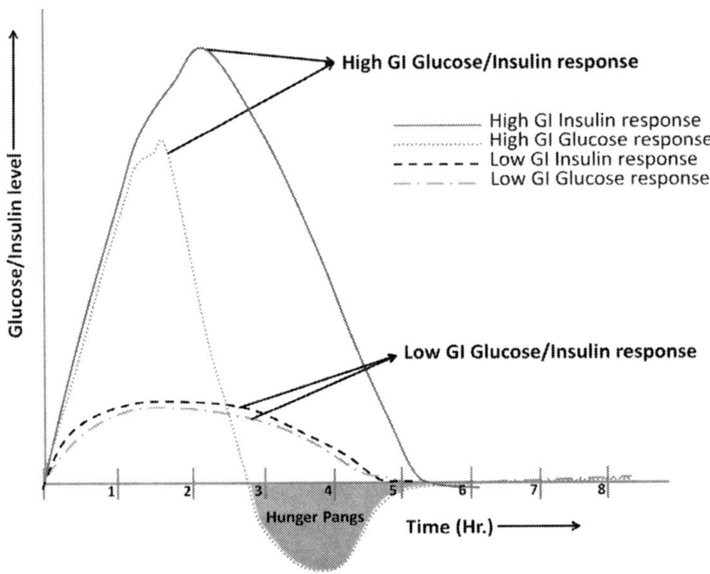

Figure 6: Blood glucose/insulin levels after a high-GI meal vs. after a low-GI meal

When the same process repeats itself, more insulin-driven fat storage occurs, and a pattern gets established. On the other hand, eating a low-GI meal causes blood sugar levels to rise slowly over a longer period of time, giving the pancreas ample time to respond efficiently to the sugar increase and to release just enough insulin in order to store the excess sugar. Once all excess sugar is stored, a normal blood sugar level is attained and there are no hunger pangs and feelings of low energy (Figure 6).

> It is this repeated process of insulin spikes and blood sugar "crashes" that causes weight gain over time

Carbohydrates that are easily digested and broken down in the gut cause the quick assimilation of sugar in the blood, followed by a quick insulin response leading to fat storage and hunger pangs. And when the hunger pangs occur, the person wants another quick burst of energy (typically from another high-GI meal) to bring back the sugar levels to normal. The process repeats and more fat storage occurs. It is this repeated process of insulin spikes and blood sugar "crashes" that causes weight gain over time. The schematic process is shown in Figure 7.

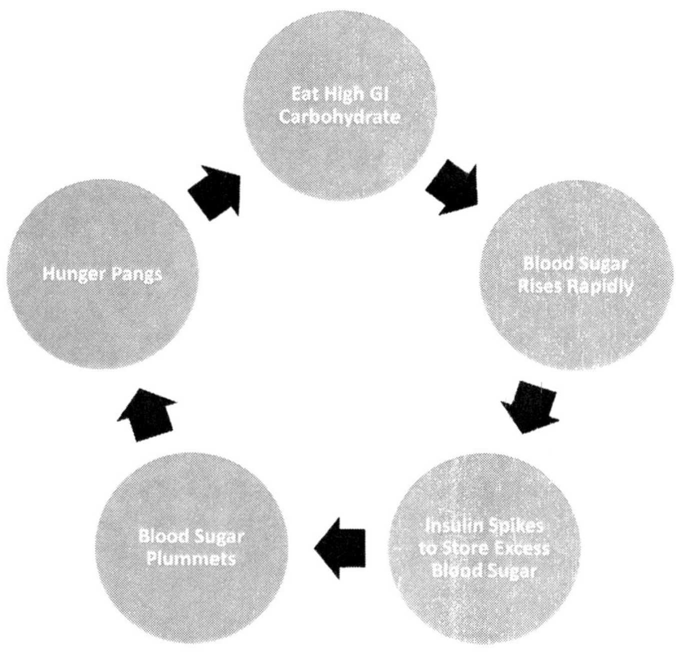

Figure 7: How chronic carbohydrate consumption drives up hunger and promotes weight gain.

To illustrate the point about GI and its effect on hunger, Dr. David Ludwig of Harvard Medical School and professor of pediatrics at Boston Hospital, conducted a study[8] where 12 adolescents were given three different kinds of breakfast of identical calories: instant oatmeal (high GI), steel cut oats (medium GI) and omelet with fruit (low GI). Their blood glucose and stress hormones were monitored following the meal. Four hours later the instant oatmeal group had the lowest blood sugar (even lower than their fasting level) inducing the greatest stress and hunger response. Basically their brain was reading "starvation" signals. The omelet group, on the other hand, had the steadiest and lowest blood sugar rise and no stress response.

For lunch all the participants were given unlimited access to tasty foods such as bagels, cream cheese, cookies etc. and it was found that the instant oatmeal group consumed 1400 calories. The steel cut oats group consumed 900 calories and the omelet group consumed 750 calories. Those 650 fewer calories between the instant oatmeal and omelet group could mean the difference between lean and obese 10 years down the road.

Carbohydrate Addiction

Many experts blame the current obesity epidemic on carbohydrate addiction. Again, Dr. David Ludwig did a test on 12 overweight men between the ages of 18-35. He gave them a high GI milkshake and a low GI milkshake and observed brain activity (using MRI) four hours after they consumed the shakes. The study[9] found that (bold emphasis is mine):

> After the men consumed the high-glycemic index milkshake, they had an initial surge in blood sugar levels, followed by a sharp crash four hours later. This decrease in blood glucose was associated with **excessive hunger** and intense activation of the nucleus accumbens, a critical brain region involved in **addictive behaviors**.
>
> Dr. Ludwig further noted that,
>
> *"Beyond reward and craving, this part of the brain is also linked to substance abuse and dependence, which raises the question as to whether certain foods might be addictive."*

This is why people who like donuts, cakes and pastries have such a hard time giving them up. And in fact, it's not just the sweet stuff that can be addictive, but any carbohydrate that's easily digested is equally addictive. Potatoes, rice, and white bread are equally addictive as they have a GI as high as or higher than ordinary table sugar.

The Dangers of Visceral Fat

In the previous sections, we saw how insulin resistance promotes the accumulation of visceral fat in the midsection. At this point, it's important to realize the threat visceral fat poses to our health.

Visceral fat is a special kind of fat. It's different from the subcutaneous fat found around your thighs, face, hips, and butt, which simply act as energy reserves. Visceral fat is active fat. Visceral fat is deadly fat. It is literally a hormone factory producing its own unique blend of inflammatory molecules such as interleukin (IL-6), tumor necrosis factor (TNF-α), resistin, and macrophage chemoattractant protein-1 that drain directly into the liver and are then circulated all around the body. These substances spell bad news for your health.

In a study[10], researchers looked at blood samples from the portal vein that drains blood from visceral fat directly into the liver of extremely obese subjects during gastric bypass surgery and found that concentrations of these inflammatory molecules were 50% greater than in blood in the other arteries. This means visceral fat is not just associated with systemic inflammation but also contributes to it. More information on inflammation and its relation to modern chronic disease can be found in Appendix G.

Not only is a bigger midsection unsightly, but it is also a bigger health hazard compared to fat found elsewhere around the body

Researchers now realize that systemic inflammation plays a key role in the progression of almost every chronic lifestyle disease such as diabetes, heart disease, Alzheimer's[11], Parkinson's, and other neurodegenerative disorders[12]. This is why doctors now find that waist-to-hip ratio, which measures the amount of visceral fat more accurately than Body Mass Index (another obesity metric), is a better predictor of risk for these chronic lifestyle diseases.

In one word, visceral fat is DANGEROUS to your health.

Not only is a bigger midsection unsightly, but it is also a bigger health hazard compared to fat found elsewhere around the body.

What's more, visceral fat is directly correlated to the production of estrogen in both males and females. This increases the risk for breast cancer in women[13], since estrogen is a known breast cell proliferator. It also causes gynecomastia or "man breasts" in obese males.

Insulin Driven Fat Storage-A Departing Shot

Figure 8, below, is a striking example of how insulin promotes fat storage. It shows a 22-year-old diabetic male who has been taking insulin injections in his thighs for the past two years. In the areas where insulin is injected, there are local areas of fat deposits, also known as insulin-induced lipohypertrophy. The areas in his thighs where insulin concentration is the highest—the point of injection—end up storing excess fat. This should serve as direct (and somewhat shocking) evidence that shows how fat storage is affected by the presence and action of insulin.

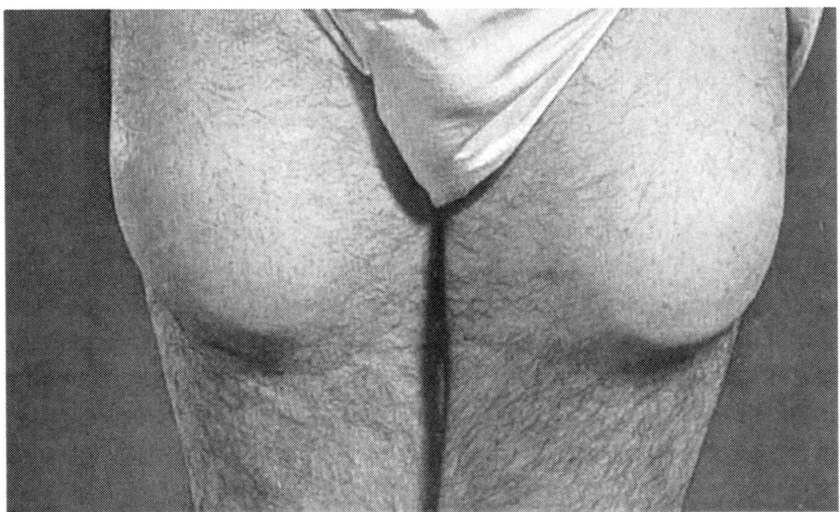

Figure 8: Insulin lipohypertrophy. (Source M. A. Papadakis, S. J. McPhee, M. W. Rabow: Current medical diagnosis and treatment 2016, 55th edition, Copyright © McGraw-Hill Education.)

CHAPTER 3

How Hunger is Controlled

"Hunger knows no friend but its feeder."

Aristophanes

In this chapter, you will learn:

- How hormones control our hunger and metabolism.
- How a shift in the hormonal balance makes our bodies efficient at storing fat.
- Why weight gain is not the consequence of gluttony and lethargy but rather the cause.

Leptin and Ghrelin: The Yin and Yang of Hunger and Metabolism

Nature relies on *homeostasis* to maintain the delicate balance that supports life. When this balance shifts dramatically, disease and often obesity take root.

This same principle applies to hunger and satiety, fat gain and fat loss. In a healthy body, one hormone acts to stimulate hunger; after you've eaten a meal, another hormone acts to suppress the hunger. The same thing applies to the metabolism of fat. One

> Leptin is the hunger satisfaction hormone that naturally inhibits hunger

hormone causes your body to store fat, and the opposing force of another hormone makes your body burn fat. This is how your body maintains a certain weight.

The two hormones, the yin and the yang of hunger and metabolism, are leptin and ghrelin. Leptin is the hunger satisfaction hormone that naturally inhibits hunger when we've had enough to eat. Leptin is secreted in the fat (adipose) tissue and it relays to the brain the status of energy (body fat) reserves in the body. Essentially, leptin sends a message to our brain, specifically the hypothalamus, to stop eating when we have had enough to eat.

The hypothalamus is in charge of all homeostatic systems in the body (thirst, body temperature, and hunger). High levels of leptin suppress hunger and boost metabolism. Ghrelin, the opposing hormone, is secreted in our gut and is often called the hunger hormone. Ghrelin also works on the receptors in the hypothalamus but has the exact opposite effect of leptin.

While leptin tells the brain that we have enough stored energy (body fat), ghrelin informs the brain that the stomach is empty. The gurgling you hear when you have an empty stomach is ghrelin at work.

Leptin: Master Key for Regulating Weight Set-point

Leptin is the second main character in our story of metabolism and weight regulation. Leptin plays a fundamentally more important role than insulin in regulating body fat levels. It works to restore long-term energy balance in the body by controlling the amount of body fat that can be stored at any given time. Based on leptin's signal, the brain decides whether to ramp up hunger and suppress metabolism (switch to weight gain mode) or to suppress hunger and ramp up metabolism (switch to weight loss mode). This is how leptin controls your weight set-point. Ghrelin, on the other hand, only acts in the short term (between meals).

In other words, leptin is the master hormone that controls how much body fat you will have! If insulin is the (sugar) Police of metabolism town, leptin is the Mayor!

In order to lose weight, you have to understand and actively work to change the leptin levels in your body.

Since leptin is the key to our problem, let's take a closer look at this fascinating hormone.

Leptin (Greek *leptos,* meaning thin) was recently discovered (in 1990) by Jeffrey Friedman et al., after they isolated a gene in a type of mice with a specific genetic mutation that made the mice eat voraciously and be massively obese (three times the normal mouse's weight). Prior to leptin's discovery, it was thought that body weight was something that could be controlled at will by varying food intake; hence the "*eat less*" recommendation to lose weight. Leptin's discovery changed that.

After leptin was discovered, researchers realized that there was a robust system in the body to tightly regulate food intake and metabolism, and that body weight can't be changed at will[14]. Friedman, in his landmark paper titled "*Modern science versus the stigma of obesity,*" showed why the simplistic notion of eating less to lose weight is counteracted by the powerful evolutionary forces within the body that maintain bodyweight within a narrow range[15]. He basically showed that the obese are not obese simply because they eat more.

The mechanism of how leptin works is beyond the scope of this book, but it is sufficient to understand that when leptin increases, hunger is suppressed and metabolism or activity level is boosted, and this favors body fat loss (arrow to the left in Figure 9). When leptin falls (or ghrelin increases), we feel intense hunger and metabolism is suppressed, and this favors body fat gain (arrow to the right in Figure 9). As long as they are working in unison, there is homeostasis and weight is maintained (center arrow in Figure 9). When the balance shifts in favor of one or the other, weight gain or weight loss occurs. A caveat to Figure 9 is that this picture is representative of a normal healthy person.

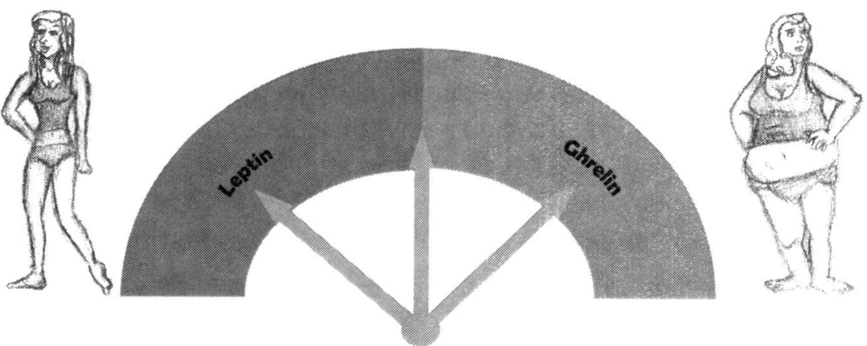

Figure 9: Leptin and ghrelin and how weight loss is affected.

How Leptin and Insulin Work Together

Leptin, along with insulin, forms what researchers refer to as the Adipoinsular axis[16], a process by which insulin stimulates the production of leptin in the fat tissue[17] and leptin inhibits the production of insulin in the pancreas[18]. What this means, in simple terms, is that insulin and leptin form a regulating feedback mechanism that guards against overeating and obesity.

Here's how the cycle works in a healthy person:

When you don't eat or when you exercise, your blood sugar levels decline. As a result, insulin (and leptin) levels start dropping. This relays to the brain a message that the energy reserves are depleting. The brain then drives up hunger and suppresses metabolism, so you'll eat and conserve stored body fat. The carbohydrates in the food you eat increase your insulin levels. The rising insulin (and the resultant fat storage) then stimulates the production of leptin. The rising levels of leptin relay to the brain a message that the energy reserves are filling up and that you have eaten enough. The brain then suppresses hunger and boosts metabolism so that the energy reserves are maintained at a set level. This built-in regulation in our body guards against uncontrolled eating and weight gain.

The Obese Have High Levels of Leptin

Since leptin is produced in the adipose tissue, the more body fat you have, the more leptin is produced. A high level of leptin suppresses hunger and boosts metabolism. By this logic, it would seem that an obese person would be less hungry and have a higher metabolic rate, to burn off the extra fat reserves. In reality, the exact opposite is observed. The obese have a bigger appetite and they have a slow metabolism, so they don't burn fat easily. In other words, they **overeat** and they are **lethargic**.

According to Dr. Robert H. Lustig, the world's foremost authority on Leptin and the author of New York Times bestseller *Fat Chance*, this apparent contradiction can be explained by the phenomena of **leptin resistance**, which occurs when leptin levels are chronically high. Chronic high-GI carbohydrate consumption keeps insulin and leptin levels high. When this happens, the leptin sensors in the brain become desensitized because they are constantly bombarded with leptin. It's like getting desensitized to traffic

insulin and leptin form a regulating feedback mechanism that guards against overeating and obesity.

noises if you live on a busy street. The brain essentially becomes deaf to leptin's signals. So even though there is plenty of leptin circulating in the body the brain senses "starvation." As a result, the hunger impulse stays high and metabolism (or activity level) stays suppressed even after the person has eaten enough and has plenty of stored body fat!

How the Weight Set-point Moves to Cause Obesity

In a healthy body, the initial leptin sensitivity is at a certain level and the body maintains a certain weight set-point based on it. Experts call this the *leptin threshold*. If your *leptin threshold* is set too low your brain is satisfied easily and keeps your hunger at bay and your metabolism (or activity level) high. In that case, no matter how much you eat your body will burn it off with a high metabolism. You will have trouble overeating and you certainly won't be able to sit sedentary for too long. In other words you will have trouble gaining weight. On the other hand if your *leptin threshold* is set too high you will tend to be a voracious eater with not much energy to do any physical task. In other words you will have trouble losing weight. In an ideal world you are gifted with a certain *leptin threshold* based you your genetic makeup and it stays fairly constant over the years. However, in a real world situation this rarely happens. The drastic changes that have happened to our diets in the past few decades have pushed our *leptin threshold* up. Let's take a closer look.

When the bulk of a person's diet consists of carbohydrates, especially the high GI kind, insulin, and as a consequence of that, leptin levels rise. The problem happens when a pattern of high (GI) carbohydrate consumption is established, leading to chronically high levels of insulin and leptin. Over a period of years, this pattern of eating causes insulin and leptin resistance. When this happens the brain becomes deaf to leptins signal and more leptin has to be released in order to attain the same "satiety" level and in order to keep the same metabolism level. Essentially your *leptin threshold* creeps up higher!

As a result, even though you have accumulated enough body fat and even though you have eaten enough calories, the brain perceives "*starvation*" and keeps ramping up hunger and suppressing activity level (metabolism) such that body fat is preserved. The brain wants you to eat more so you can gain more fat and release even more leptin in order to satisfy the brain. This is the vicious positive feedback cycle that pushes the weight set-point to move toward increasing adiposity (fat accumulation).

over reliance on easily processed carbohydrates to provide the bulk of our energy needs pushes our body's leptin threshold towards increasing adiposity

The longer the pattern of carbohydrate consumption the higher the leptin-resistance. The higher the leptin resistance the higher the *leptin threshold* to accumulate body fat. This is how obesity takes root. Moving the weight set-point to favor weight gain is a 3-step process shown in the schematic in Figure 10.

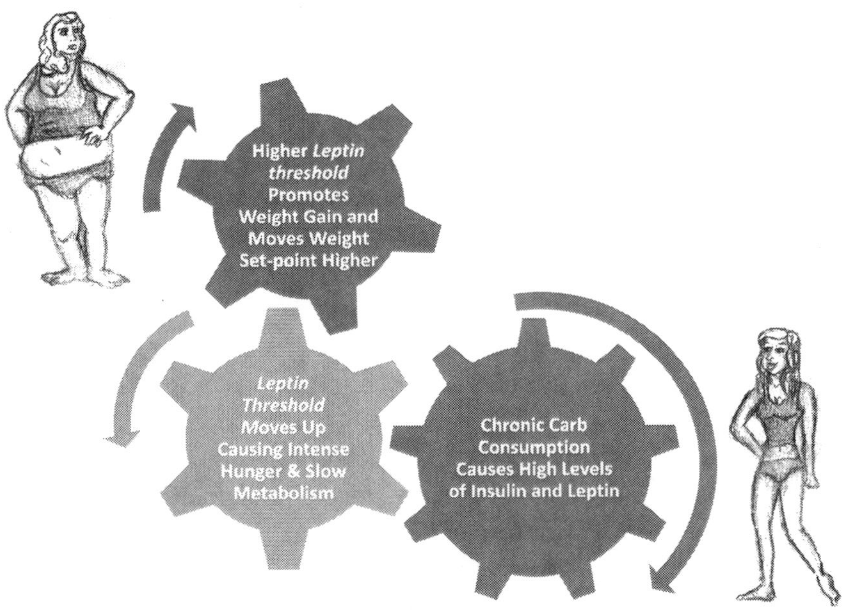

Figure 10: How chronic carbohydrate consumption causes the weight set-point to move toward increasing weight gain.

Bottom-line is this: over reliance on easily processed carbohydrates to provide the bulk of our energy needs pushes our body's *leptin threshold* towards increasing adiposity. The result is constant hunger, lethargy and weight gain!

Leptin Sensitivity is The Key to Weight Loss

It's obvious that the solution to this problem is to reverse leptin resistance. Or in other words, to sensitize the brain to leptin's signals. The only way that is possible is by getting our insulin levels lower, which will also drive down the leptin levels. Over time, the low levels of leptin will re-sensitize the brain. Once that happens, the brain will be able to listen to leptin's signal and suppress hunger and boost metabolism. Basically, the pattern that moved the weight set-point toward increasing weight gain has to be reversed to move the weight set-point back toward losing weight.

The key strategy to lowering insulin and leptin—and thus reducing body fat—is to restrict carbohydrates

Once again, according to Dr. Lustig:

> *"We have shown that insulin is the primary cause of leptin resistance. So lowering insulin makes you leptin sensitive, so that you can lose weight."*

The key strategy to lowering insulin and leptin—and thus reducing body fat—is to restrict carbohydrates and replace those calories with protein and healthy fats. This lowers leptin levels and re-sensitizes your brain to the effect of leptin. Once you are re-sensitized, your body can easily switch into fat-burning mode (Figure 11).

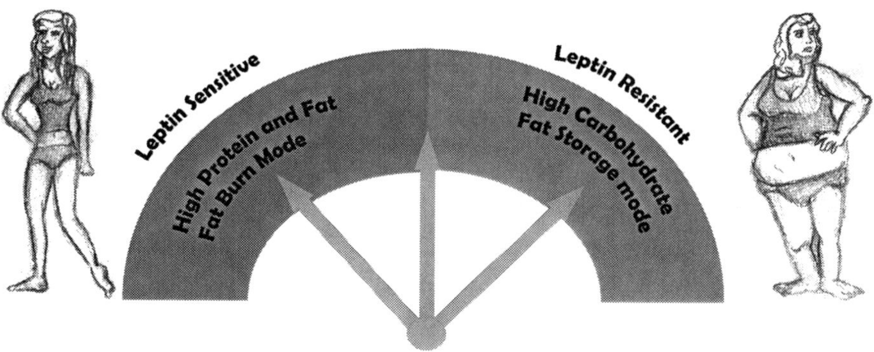

Figure 11: How a diet of protein and fat causes leptin sensitivity and weight loss.

Obesity: Cause or Consequence?

Let's revisit the question I put forth in the Introduction: is it because we overeat and become lazy that we gain weight? Or is it because our body's hormonal state wants us to gain weight, making us hungry and lazy in the process?

We have seen so far how the USDA high-carbohydrate diet makes our bodies extremely efficient at storing body fat. The moment we eat, we start the insulin-driven weight gain and all the energy from our food is sequestered in the fat cells. Once this happens, we are left with no energy to meet our daily needs. As a result, we get hungry and lethargic.

Again, Dr. David S. Ludwig of Harvard Medical School makes a claim in his paper "*Increasing Adiposity: Consequence or Cause of Overeating?*"[19] that turns the age-old calorie-in-calorie-out hypothesis of weight gain on its head. He proposes that the reason we overeat is because our bodies sequester all the food calories as body fat, putting our bodies in a constant energy deficit mode. This causes feelings of intense hunger and lethargy.

hunger and lethargy are not the cause of weight gain but rather a consequence of weight gain

Our bodies now rely instead on excess food intake to meet our daily energy needs. At this stage, it's nearly impossible to make the body burn its stored fat reserves even if we completely starve ourselves. What happens instead is that the body's metabolism comes to a screeching halt and the person ceases all activity and becomes lethargic, but still is unable to lose fat.

Therefore, he says, hunger and lethargy are not the cause of weight gain but rather a consequence of weight gain.

Case in Point: Federal Economic Stimulus

Let me give an example: The Federal Reserve, in 2008, provided an economic stimulus to the banks in excess of billions of dollars in hopes that the money would trickle down to the consumers and invigorate the sluggish economy. But it did nothing. The economy still stayed sluggish and the Federal Reserve continued to pump more stimulus dollars into the economy.

The reason the stimulus dollars didn't invigorate the economy was because the banks held on to the stimulus dollars and never put them back into the system (as consumer loans). So the economy continued to be sluggish requiring more money to be fed into the economy. There was nothing wrong with the economy. It was the fact that the stimulus money was immediately being sequestered by the banks that made the economy sluggish.

Likewise, in the case of an obese person, when the person eats food (economic stimulus) the calories (dollars) that would otherwise be available for daily activity (consumer economy) are quickly sequestered in fat cells (banks). As a result of this, the person gets lethargic (sluggish economy) and stays hungry (needing more stimulus dollars).

Case in Point: Adolescents and Growth Spurts

Another good example is an adolescent going through puberty. Ever notice how a teenager is always hungry and too lazy to get out of bed in the morning? He/she has to be prodded to do even the simplest household chores and can never seem to have enough food. Teenagers also gain considerable muscle and bone mass during this period. Is all this growth caused from overeating and lethargy? Or is the lethargy and overeating due to this growth? Let's find out.

The human body goes through hormonal changes that create the groundwork for the growth spurts that happen during puberty. The bones and muscles need all the energy to support this rapid growth; the body achieves this by increasing hunger and suppressing metabolism to conserve calories. This causes the teenager to overeat and be lazy. So the teenager going through a growth spurt is not growing as a consequence of overeating and laziness. The growth spurt is causing the overeating and laziness.

Likewise, in the case of leptin resistance: the proclivity of the body to gain weight causes overeating and lethargy and not the other way around. Remove the leptin resistance and the hunger and lethargy will disappear and weight will be lost!

The answer to my initial question is that the obese are not obese because they overeat and are lazy, but because their body is so efficient at storing fat it makes them overeat and become lazy! This new understanding of the cause and effect of weight gain will help us reverse the conditions that led to it in the first place.

Size Doesn't Matter

While size might matter in the bedroom, when it comes to the dining table the size of your plate doesn't matter. What really matters is what's on it.

Easily digested processed carbohydrates tend to switch your body into storage mode. Natural wholesome foods full of healthy fats and fiber keep your body in fuel-burning mode so you continue to use the fuel from food instead of storing it (and asking for more food).

We have natural checks and balances built into our body to guard against overeating and starvation. The leptin feedback system is meant to protect us from gaining weight or wasting away, but the assault of modern processed foods and the misinformation we are fed has destroyed this delicate balance and put us into a sick, fattened state.

Dr. David Ludwig suggests abandoning the calorie-centric view of obesity and focusing instead on changing the dietary composition to best facilitate long-term weight loss.

The human body is not a simple mechanical system. The interaction of various macronutrients within our body is much more complex for weight gain and loss to be explained by the simplistic model proposed by the calories in/calories out hypothesis. This is why it isn't able to explain our growing waistlines and our tipping scales in spite of being a calorie-counting society.

Is Leptin Resistance a Disease?

Other than a few leading researchers, most doctors don't identify leptin resistance as an ailment or disease that needs treatment, even though it is at the root of a host of metabolic disorders that eventually cause obesity, type II diabetes, cardiovascular disease, and many other chronic ailments. Leptin resistance is not something that's tested for.

Society as a whole (including most doctors) ascribes personal responsibility for someone being obese. They blame the obese person for lacking willpower to eat less and exercise more. But this doesn't explain the growing number of overweight infants, because no infant intentionally wants to overeat and be lazy. Obesity has its roots in hormonal causes and blaming personal responsibility isn't going to address the problem.

The good news, though, is that these hormonal imbalances can easily be reversed with the right diet and lifestyle. By doing so, the same hormonal forces that cause you to gain weight can also be used to help you lose weight effortlessly, which is the practical subject of Part 2.

CHAPTER 4

How Stress Promotes Weight Gain

"You don't get ulcers from what you eat. You get them from what's eating you."

Vicki Baum

In this chapter, you will see:

- How stress promotes (visceral) belly fat.
- Why a person under stress tends to gravitate toward easy carbohydrate fixes.

Any discussion about weight gain is incomplete without a discussion of stress and how it contributes to weight gain. How many times have you reached for the vending machine when you are worried about a project report and eaten something sugary? Sounds familiar, doesn't it? We all have been under stress at various times in our lives, whether it is related to money or family problems or just from being stuck in bad traffic.

At a fundamental level, what is stress?

It is any external or internal state of disharmony that challenges either our physical or emotional integrity. Stress causes a cascade of hormonal response from our hypothalamus, pituitary, and adrenal glands, collectively known as the HPA Axis. This results in the release of two distinct hormones in our body: adrenalin and cortisol. These are responses to two types of stresses: short-term momentary stress, and long-term subliminal stress.

The first, adrenalin, is responsible for fight-or-flight response during times of impending calamity. Someone pointing a gun to your head in a dark alleyway will cause the release of adrenalin, which prepares you to either fight or run away from the stressor (flight). This causes your heart rate and blood pressure to go up, your liver to quickly release blood sugar to power the brain and muscles for a quick reaction, your pupils to dilate so that more light can enter your eyes for better visibility, etc. But this type of stress is momentary and doesn't do much to our long-term health.

> the stress hormone cortisol takes fat from our arms and legs and stores it as dangerous visceral fat

The second type of stress is the slow, nagging stress of daily life. Daily stress is an inseparable part of our lives. In the daily hustle and bustle, we are always scrambling to compress more and more work into the twenty-four hours we have. The stress of a looming deadline, the stress of paying bills, the stress of taxes, the stress of daily traffic are all examples of overt stresses that we all experience every now and then. Another variant of this stress is one that works at a deeper subliminal level, like anxiety and depression.

This slow nagging stress of daily life and other subliminal stresses cause the release of the second stress hormone, cortisol. Cortisol works in the same way as adrenalin, but over a longer period of time. Cortisol also causes the liver to churn out sugar in order to power the brain. With chronic stress, the cortisol levels constantly stay high, causing your blood sugar to be high all the time. This in turn causes your insulin and leptin levels to stay high as well. This again pushes your insulin/leptin feedback mechanism out of control, causing weight gain.

In a healthy person, the initial emotional stress causes a rise in insulin and leptin levels[20] via cortisol and creates the loss of appetite from being leptin sensitive, but over time, as leptin and insulin resistance sets in, the appetite grows, and people reach out for the easy carbohydrate fix.

How Stress Promotes Visceral Fat

Rather than causing a net weight gain, cortisol causes weight redistribution. A simple explanation of the mechanism is that cortisol commands the peripheral fat cells, located in our arms and legs, to release triglycerides into the bloodstream. These triglycerides are then converted to blood sugar (in the liver) and released into the bloodstream. Now insulin comes into play and starts storing this excess sugar. Since visceral fat has a higher sensitivity to insulin compared to fat cells in other parts of our body, this excess sugar ends up as stored belly fat. Essentially, the stress hormone cortisol takes fat from our arms and legs and stores it as dangerous visceral fat[21].

An extreme example of this is Cushing's disease (name after Dr. Harvey Cushing, who was the first person to describe it) where, due to abnormalities of the pituitary gland, excess cortisol is produced in the body. The physical characteristics of this disease show an increased weight gain in the midsection, along with high blood pressure, diabetes, and increased susceptibility to heart disease. All the same symptoms of obesity related diseases!

Case in Point: Stress in Immigrants

Researchers have done extensive studies on immigrants living in foreign lands and have shown that they have high levels of this chronic stress. Studies done on native populations that are displaced during times of civil strife or war[22] have also shown high incidence of this type of stress. The stress of social dislocation (being in a foreign land), cultural alienation, socioeconomic stress, depression and anxiety are all examples of subliminal stresses that are faced by these populations and manifest itself in higher rates of heart disease, metabolic syndrome and type II diabetes.

In a large study done from 1978 through 1985, data from about 13,000 participants in Northern California showed that (Asian) Indians have four times more hospitalizations from coronary artery disease (CAD) than whites and six times higher than Chinese (Figure 12)[23].

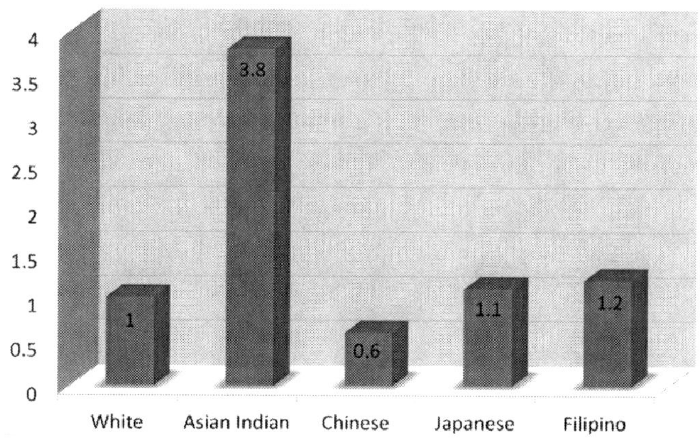

Figure 12: Relative rates of hospitalizations for CAD in northern California for various ethnicities (Courtesy of http://www.cadiresearch.org).

Like immigrant Indians, Japanese immigrants living in the United States have a higher mortality rate from heart disease than those living in Japan[24]. Traditionally, the Japanese were believed to have superior genetics with respect to heart disease (since Japan has the highest number of centenarians alive) but all this genetic superiority disappears when they start living abroad, even as they continue to consume their traditional diet. This phenomenon is true for immigrants all over the globe.

The same has been found true of Indian immigrants living in Singapore compared to Singapore natives. A study done in the 1990[25] found:

> *"...the higher mortality from ischemic heart disease found in Indians in Singapore cannot be explained by the major risk factors of cigarette smoking, blood pressure and serum cholesterol."*

Compared to Singapore natives, the immigrants smoked less, had lower blood pressure and cholesterol, and yet—counterintuitively—their mortality rate was higher. The same study also noted that the immigrants had a higher incidence of diabetes.

A meta-analysis of 58 studies (published between 1986 and 2008) relating to deaths from myocardial infarction (MI) among first-generation immigrant populations worldwide found that[26]:

> *"...there was an overall trend for increasing risk of MI among immigrants worldwide."*

Another meta-analysis of 23 studies of immigrant populations in Australia sought the answer to this question: Is being an immigrant a heart disease risk factor? They concluded[27] that:

> *"...higher prevalence of cardiovascular disease was found among Middle Eastern, South Asian and some European immigrants."*

In another remarkable study done in London, 364 participants were divided into two groups where one group was first generation immigrants living in London and the other group was their siblings living in Punjab. This eliminated any genetic or hereditary factors from corrupting the results. It was found that the London immigrants had higher Body Mass Index, blood pressure and insulin resistance compared to their siblings in India, putting them at a higher risk of heart disease[28].

The same is true for Bangladeshis living in London, who, in spite of having lower cholesterol, eating a lower-fat diet, and smoking less, were found to have higher mortality rate from heart disease compared to the English residents of London[29].

Stress and Comfort foods

Long-term chronic stress can lead to increased visceral fat and put us at a risk for a great many chronic diseases. Now let's see how stress affects our eating patterns.

It's been found that stress suppresses appetite in the short term and that is because Cortisol has been shown to increase leptin production[30]. This has the effect of suppressing your appetite (remember the more leptin you have, the less hungry you are). But in the long term, cortisol induced leptin increase leads to leptin resistance and a resultant appetite increase[31]. This has been especially found true for women where high cortisol levels cause stress-induced eating[32]. Psychological stress has also shown to affect an increase in the secretion of the hunger hormone ghrelin, which promotes hunger and reduced metabolic rate[33].

We saw in Chapter 2 how certain easily-digested carbohydrates can be addictive by activating the brain centers that are involved in addictive behaviors. These same foods also inhibit activity in parts of brain that produce and process stress and related emotions.

Two of the most important neurotransmitters, serotonin and dopamine induce sleep and produce a calming effect on the brain. The amino acids tryptophan and tyrosine are the precursors that form serotonin and dopamine in the brain. Dr. Richard Wurtman and Dr. John D. Fernstrom of the Department of Nutrition and Food Science at MIT found that eating a carbohydrate-rich meal and the resultant insulin spike reduce the levels of other competing amino acids leaving tryptophan and tyrosine available for the production of serotonin and dopamine[34]. This explains why you feel the urge to reach for a jelly-filled donut or a Twinkie right before a big exam or an important presentation, because it calms you down and makes you feel good.

in the long term, cortisol induced leptin increase leads to leptin resistance

Other studies done at Tufts University School of Medicine and Temple University reported that tryptophan can be used to treat mild insomnia and to combat pain without any adverse side effects[35] So the term "comfort foods" is not a mere metaphor but has actual physiological significance[36].

Stress and the Effect of Food Texture

Stress has also shown to increase food intake in the absence of hunger, especially foods that are crisp in texture and give you fullness of taste such as something that quickly melts in your mouth and coats your taste buds[37].

psychological stress and obesity form a positive feedback cycle that feed off each other in a downward spiral of weight gain

Potato chips (crispy) and cream-filled Twinkies (melt in your mouth) come to mind. The best comfort foods are those that incorporate all three elements of taste, i.e., sweetness with a crispy outer layer and a melt-in-your-mouth inner core, such as cream-filled pastry shells or crème brûlée or deep fried ice cream. It shouldn't surprise you to know that the processed food industry spends millions of dollars developing these exact taste attributes in packaged snacks.

The other reason these taste attributes work against you is that since they quickly melt in your mouth and pass through to your gut, they don't give the leptin feedback system ample time to respond. So while you are binging on the extra calories, your brain still thinks it hasn't had enough calories and you continue to eat. Under stress, people are drawn to these types of high energy density (but zero nutritional value) foods that lead to rapid weight gain, especially in the midsection.

The flip side of the coin is that obesity has shown to induce depression and anxiety in adolescents and young adults via lack of self-esteem, which then draws them toward "comfort" foods[38]. So psychological stress and obesity form a positive feedback cycle that feed off each other in a downward spiral of weight gain.

Be a Conscious Eater

The only way to stop this downward spiral is to be a conscious eater. If you are depressed or anxious and want to reach out to the vending machine, ask yourself if you are really hungry or if you are just doing this to escape the feeling of depression and anxiety?

Studies have also shown the less you eat junk food the less you crave for it. So you stop yourself from eating junk food once and it gets easier the next time and so on and so forth. Eventually you build enough momentum and willpower that you will be able to walk past the vending machine without even thinking about it.

When it comes to stress and worrying, remember what the Dalai Lama said:

“If a problem is fixable, if a situation is such that you can do something about it, then there is no need to worry. If it’s not fixable, then there is no help in worrying. There is no benefit in worrying whatsoever.”

CHAPTER 5

Exercise and Weight Loss

"Exercise for health, NOT weight loss."

Dr. Spencer Nadolsky

In this chapter, you will learn:

- Why vigorous exercising cannot help you lose weight in the long run
- Why being active and exercising moderately is best, for sustained weight loss

This chapter brings us to the "exercise more" part of the oft-heard advice "eat less and exercise more." Weight loss conjures up images of sweaty bodies in pain, huffing and puffing their way to skinny-land. The fitness industry sells us the image of perfect bodies with chiseled abs, toned legs, and size zero clothes. And that image works well for fitness industry profits. Sadly, it does nothing to make us any leaner.

According to the International Health, Racquet & Sportsclub Association (IHRSA), the annual gym memberships in the US has grown to $21.8 billion; about 51.2 million Americans are members of gyms and health clubs[39]. Yet as a society, we seem to be getting fatter and sicker. So something doesn't add up.

In the beginning of the book, I alluded to the exercise aspect of weight loss and how it's ineffective at losing weight in the long run due to powerful homeostatic mechanisms at work that are striving to maintain your bodyweight set-point. In this chapter, I'll dispel the myth that exercise is mandatory in order to lose weight.

Doing the Numbers: Why Exercise-related Calorie Loss is Not Enough to Lose Weight.

One gram of fat contains nine calories. This means one pound of fat contains about 3,900 calories. One hour of jogging at a moderate pace burns about 500-600 calories. To lose just a pound of fat you will have to jog for about seven hours. You can quickly see the calories burned doing exercise are inefficient at burning excess body fat, not to mention the additional hunger that you have to ward off in order to prevent yourself from eating the lost calories. Plus, not everyone can jog or exercise due to physical or time constraints.

Exercising for weight loss is akin to sweating for water loss

Exercising for weight loss is akin to sweating for water loss. Research has shown that physical exercise lowers insulin and leptin levels[40]. This stimulates hunger, and if you follow your "natural instinct" and eat until you are satisfied, you would eat about the same number of extra calories that you burned exercising. No weight loss would occur. This is similar to drinking more water after sweating.

The reason most people see weight loss from exercise is because they simultaneously give up other "unhealthy" eating habits. For example, after a one-hour jog, it's likely you will turn down that donut or candy bar and eat a celery stick or a carrot or a salad instead. You will also exert willpower to limit your calorie intake, in line with the "eat less, exercise more" dictum. That's the real reason you'll lose weight, and not because you are exercising. In fact, if you continued your "usual" eating habits, exercise might actually make you gain weight. This is because exercise will stimulate some muscle growth (a good thing) and muscle is denser than fat.

Studies comparing the physical activity levels and calorie intakes of lumberjacks to tailors, found that the strenuous physical demands on lumberjacks caused them to eat twice the number of calories (5000 calories/day) compared to tailors (2500 calories/day). Yet the lumberjacks were no leaner than the tailors. In fact, if anything, the lumberjacks weighed more than the tailors. Study after study has come to the same conclusion and that is: the more demanding the physical activity, the more it stimulates hunger.

In a more recent CUT-IT[C](randomized) trial published in 2014[41], two groups of people were separated into an "exercise more" group (aerobic interval training) and an "eat less" group (low-energy diet). After 10-14 weeks, it was found that the "eat less" group lost about 10% body weight compared to the exercising group that lost only 1.6% bodyweight. Not too convincing evidence in favor of exercising for weight loss.

In fact, Russell Wilder, an obesity expert from the Mayo Clinic in 1932, noted that his "fat patients lost more weight with bed rest," while "unusually strenuous physical exercise slows the rate of weight loss."

The "eat less and exercise more" recommendation we hear from the experts disregards the important link between eating and exercising, and that is "hunger." And hunger doesn't allow that to work, at least not in the long run. The more you exercise, the hungrier you get, period!

Once again, Dr. David Ludwig, director of the New Balance Foundation Obesity Prevention Center at Boston Children's Hospital, writes, "If you just try to eat less and exercise more, most people will lose that battle. Metabolism wins."

The complex relationship between exercise and weight loss cannot be explained by a simple thermodynamic model of calories in/calories out. Weight loss is more about eating the right foods in the right quantities than just exercising more (and eating less).

The "eat less and exercise more" recommendation we hear from the experts disregards the important link between eating and exercising, and that is "hunger."

What Exercise is Good For

Exercise, if done right, however, has many other benefits besides weight loss. Exercise reduces stress, delays osteoporosis, reduces the risk of heart disease and other chronic conditions, and the list goes on and on. Everyone who can exercise should do so, but realize that just because you have worked out for an hour in the gym doesn't mean you will weigh any less, unless of course you eat smart at the same time.

I suggest, "Eat smart for weight loss and exercise for wellness."

C Copenhagen study of overweight patients with coronary artery disease undergoing low energy diet or interval training: the randomized CUT-IT trial

How Long-term Endurance Exercise Sabotages Your Weight Loss

Exercise has its benefits. Low to moderate intensity exercise improves mood, reduces stress, and lowers your risk for many chronic diseases. But too much exercise can be harmful as well. As with anything in life, there is a point of marginal returns; beyond a certain point, you reach a point of negative returns. Similarly, with exercise when overdone, you reach a point of negative returns.

Exercise causes an increase in hunger that makes "eating less" difficult. But beyond increasing hunger, exercise causes physical stress, and like any other external stress, it also causes the production of cortisol. Long duration exercise that lasts over an hour overproduces cortisol[42] and cortisol is a known catabolic agent (meaning, it breaks down muscle and bone tissue). Furthermore, we have seen that cortisol overproduction spells bad news for our leptin sensitivity, which makes it hard for us to lose weight.

> moderate to mild exercise is more effective for losing weight than prolonged intense exercise

Studies show that moderate to mild exercise is more effective for losing weight than prolonged intense exercise, due to excess cortisol production in the latter case. In one study[43], researchers measured cortisol levels in blood before and after exercise at 40%, 60%, and 80% maximum intensity and found an increase in cortisol levels by 40% and 83% for exercise at 60% and 80% intensity respectively. What was more surprising is that they found 40% intensity exercise reduced cortisol levels by 6.6%! So mild to moderate exercise was found to reduce cortisol levels. A win-win for weight loss and wellness!

Repeated exercise-induced stress adapts our body to become stronger the next time that stress is presented, provided we are fully recovered. But with long duration exercise done frequently the body isn't able to cope with exercise-induced stress and breaks down more than it can recover. So the next time you find yourself feeling like a hamster on the treadmill trying to get rid of belly fat, it may be time to step off the treadmill and take a leisurely walk instead.

The Right Exercise to Lose Weight is to Stay Active

Another important concept to understand is how the Basal Metabolic Rate (BMR) plays into the effects of exercise on your body. BMR is the amount of calories the body burns at rest. This is the minimum energy required to sustain vital body functions of the heart, lungs, kidneys, pancreas, liver, brain, and skeletal muscles when you are in a rested state. Essentially, this is the minimum energy needed for you to survive. BMR comprises 60% of your daily energy expenditure budget. So 60% of the calories you consume everyday goes into keeping you alive.

What about the remaining 40%?

The remaining 40% of your energy budget is divided into energy needed to digest food and energy needed to perform daily activities. Scientists call the first, Food Thermogenesis, which takes up 10% of your daily energy budget; and the second, Activity Thermogenesis, which takes up the remaining 30%. Activity Thermogenesis can be further divided into categories of exercise (like running or weight training) and non-exercise (climbing stairs, taking the bus, brushing teeth, cleaning dishes, fidgeting, doing laundry, etc.). For a sedentary person who does no formal exercise, all the activity energy expenditure will come from non-exercise activity thermogenesis (also known as NEAT) shown in Figure 13

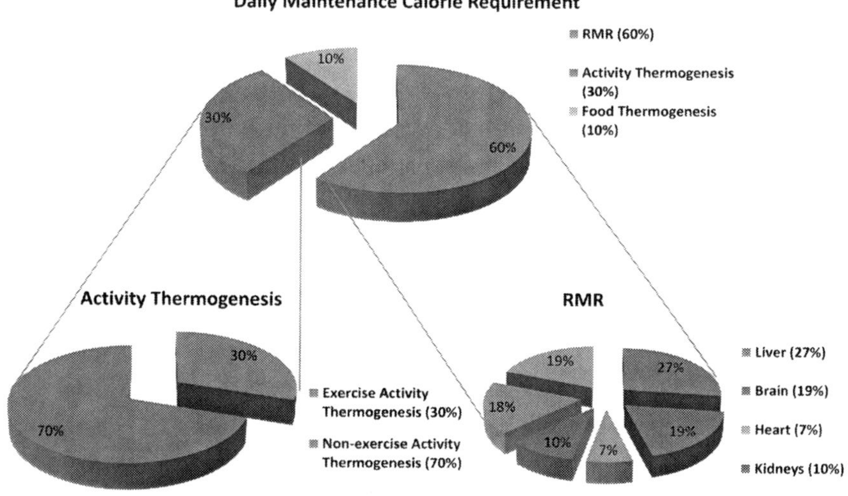

Figure 13: Daily energy expenditure budget.

Non-exercise activity thermogenesis (NEAT) burns more than twice the energy used during exercise, even for avid exercisers. This is why it's important to keep your daily NEAT energy expenditure high by staying active during the course of the day. Work around the house, do dishes, do laundry, and walk wherever possible. Don't keep a water bottle by your desk but walk to the water cooler every time you need a drink. Take the stairs whenever possible and walk around in your work area every hour or so. For weight loss, what you do outside of the gym matters more than what you do in the gym.

There is no doubt that vigorous exercise burns calories, but by the same token, it also increases hunger. And if you rely on "exercise more" to stay lean, then you are fighting a losing battle. Staying active or exercising mildly doesn't disturb your hunger/metabolism balance so it's easier to keep it up in the long run and give you the same calorie loss benefit as vigorous exercise, minus the hunger (and cortisol).

if you rely on "exercise more" to stay lean, then you are fighting a losing battle

Closing Thoughts: What We Can Learn From Centenarians

I would like to close this chapter and Part 1 with practical life lessons that we can learn from the lives of centenarians (people who live beyond the age of 100). Studies of centenarian populations show remarkable similarities, even though they come from varied backgrounds and even though some of them are lifelong smokers (and have other vices):

1) **They have well-regulated insulin levels:** they eat an unprocessed wholesome diet (both animal- and plant-based). This keeps their insulin levels well regulated (no insulin spikes). This also has the effect of keeping them leptin-sensitive.

2) **They have low stress levels:** they are mostly spiritual, which gives them a positive outlook on life. Also, they live in relatively rural places, which keeps them away from environmental pollution and big-city problems. They also live in joint families or close to their loved ones. The result of all this is that they are better able to cope with stress.

3) **They lead an active lifestyle but are not avid exercisers:** they are active on a daily basis. They work around the house or yard; they walk a lot; and they spend time playing with their grandchildren, etc. Very rarely, you will find a centenarian who is an avid exerciser.

All these common traits point to well-regulated insulin levels and high leptin sensitivity. This is why they are almost always lean and rarely obese. So the key to staying lean, healthy, and living long is:

Manage insulin, lower stress levels, and lead an active lifestyle.

Part 2 deals with putting the lessons learned into practice for effortless weight loss.

PART 2

PRACTICAL WEIGHT LOSS MADE EASY

CHAPTER 6

Eat Yourself Skinny: The Flat Belly Super Foods

"Don't eat anything your great-great grandmother wouldn't recognize as food. There are a great many food-like items in the supermarket your ancestors wouldn't recognize as food...stay away from these"

Michael Pollan

In this chapter, you will learn:

- Not all calories are the same, and why calories from some foods are better at helping you lose weight than others
- Why eating more of the right foods will make you skinnier

A Calorie is Not a Calorie: The Thermic Effect of Food

The calorie in/calorie out (CICO) hypothesis of weight loss is based on the misconception that all calories are the same regardless of their source. All calories are not equal, and it's important to understand the impact this fact has on weight gain and loss.

Fat has more than twice the number of calories compared to carbohydrates or proteins. Carbohydrates and proteins each have 4 calories per gram, while fat has 9 calories per gram. That's why fat has been seen as the culprit and taken much of the blame for making us fat.

Beyond the number of calories in a food item, the bigger issue is how those calories are processed in our body. This brings forth the concept of the "efficiency" of digesting a particular food, or what researchers like to call the "thermic effect" of food (TEF).

The "thermic effect" of food simply means that the body uses fat, carbohydrates, and proteins with varying efficiency. The digestive system itself uses a certain amount of energy to digest various foods. At a biochemical level, digestion requires certain chemical bonds to be broken and certain chemical reactions to occur in order to extract energy from food. These chemical reactions give off energy as heat. The energy given off in the process of digestion is the thermic loss from food, also known as food thermogenesis (Chapter 5, Figure 13). So not all calories from any food are 100% absorbed in the body. Part of those calories are lost as thermic heat.

by replacing carbohydrate calories with protein calories, you cut your available calories by about 25%

The estimated thermic loss from digesting carbohydrates is approximately 2%-3%. It is 6%-8% for fat, and 25%-30% for proteins[44]. This means if you ate a pure carbohydrate meal (of, say, fat-free cookies) of 2000 calories, the body would lose 2%-3% of those calories in digesting those cookies, or 40-60 calories. Essentially, your body would have about 1950 useful calories from such a meal. Compare this to a pure protein meal (of, say, lean chicken) of 2000 calories. In this case, your body would spend 25%-30% of those calories digesting the protein. Just by replacing carbohydrate calories with protein calories, you cut your available calories by about 25%. This digestive inefficiency is one of the reasons people who replace carbohydrates with protein can lose weight even though they consume the same number of total calories.

In the example above, the person eating 2000 calories of pure protein per day is getting about 500 fewer calories compared to the person eating 2000 calories of pure carbohydrate per day. That is about the number of calories burnt jogging for an hour—without jogging! Sort of like having your cake and eating it too. Even though the example given is extreme, you see the advantage of replacing some of the carbohydrates in your diet with protein.

Protein: The New Fat Burner

In terms of digestive efficiency, the body is most inefficient at digesting protein. 25% of calories from proteins are wasted in digestive thermic losses. The question is, can this thermic loss be used to our advantage to lose weight without cutting calories? You bet it can!

In a study comparing a high protein diet with a high carbohydrate diet it was found that eating a high protein diet increases the energy burnt two-fold compared to a high carbohydrate diet, 2.5 hours following the meal[45]. That's a 100% jump in your basal metabolic rate (BMR) which could prove quite useful for weight loss (Figure 14).

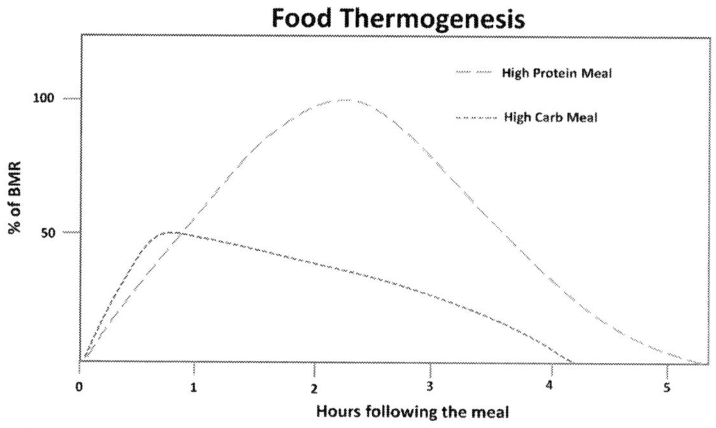

Figure 14: Percentage change in BMR following a high protein meal vs. a high carbohydrate meal.

Protein (and fat) also have a high satiety factor (meaning they are more satisfying to the palate) compared to simple carbohydrates.[46]. This is why you don't feel hungry for a few hours if you eat a cheese omelet for breakfast compared to eating a muffin or a bagel of equal calories. Not only is the muffin or bagel quickly digested (and stored away as fat) but it is also less satisfying to the brain compared to a high protein and fat cheese omelet. This has been confirmed in studies that have shown that eating a high-protein breakfast

> Adding protein to your diet not only burns additional calories in digestion, but also keeps hunger at bay in subsequent meals.

such as eggs compared to eating bread promotes weight loss by decreasing food intake in subsequent meals[47].

Adding protein to your diet not only burns additional calories in digestion, but also keeps hunger at bay in subsequent meals.

Fat: The Belly-Fat Buster

Fat has been maligned in recent decades as the biggest reason for our growing waistlines. Ever since the USDA pyramid was invented in the 1990s, fat has been relegated to the top of the pyramid in the "use sparingly" category and lumped along with sugar.

In the words of Nina Teicholz, the author of The *Big Fat Surprise: Why Butter, Meat and Cheese Belong in a Healthy Diet*:

> *"Has there ever been a more unfortunate homonym? One word means two very different things: the fat we eat and the fat on our bodies."*

The moment someone sees the word "fat" on a nutritional label, they simply assume that it's going to be stored in them. The facts about fat couldn't be farther from truth when it comes to realizing its immense healthful benefits to human health and longevity. Weight loss is just one of the benefits. Appendix D has more detailed information on fat and its health benefits for the inquisitive reader. For people who are scared of eating fat thinking that it will give them heart disease, please refer to Appendix E for more information on saturated fat and cholesterol and their relation to heart disease.

The most important thing to know (and change your mind about) is that fat is a good thing. Fat adds satiety and palatability to food. If you ever noticed how adding butter to certain foods makes them tastier and more satisfying, then you know what I am talking about. The satiety it adds to food prevents us from overeating. Fat also slows the breakdown of carbohydrates in the gut. This causes the blood sugar to rise slowly. This essentially has the effect of lowering the GI of food and of lowering insulin levels.

The three most important types of fats for the purpose of weight loss and wellness are:

1) Mono-unsaturated Fatty Acids (MUFA)
2) Medium Chain Triglycerides (MCT)
3) Omega-3 Fatty Acids

Mono-Unsaturated Fatty Acids (MUFA)

Fat refers to a combination of many fatty acid chains of varying (carbon-carbon chain) lengths. The most important one for our purpose is the Mono-Unsaturated Fatty Acid (or MUFA) that is found in seeds, nuts, olives, avocados, butter, and other animal fats.

In The New York Times bestseller *Flat Belly Diet*, author Liz Vaccariello talks about the merits of eating MUFAs to target belly fat reduction[48].

A 2008 study[49] found that people consuming a high-protein diet rich in MUFA lost 28 pounds in three months compared to people who ate the regular USDA diet. Additionally, the MUFA-rich diet improved heart health by increasing the levels of HDL (good cholesterol) and lowering triglycerides, fasting blood sugar , LDL (bad cholesterol), and blood pressure.

In another recent study, it was found that a diet rich in MUFA actually prevented the development of belly fat[50].

Medium Chain Triglycerides (MCT)

MCTs are another type of fatty acids that are abundant in certain fats like coconut oil and palm kernel oil. It's also found in sources of dairy fats like butter, milk, and cheese. Being shorter in chain length, they are relatively soluble in water and as a result, quickly absorbed in the gut. MCT is shown to be easily burned for energy and favor satiety and belly fat loss.

In a study[51] of overweight women with high abdominal obesity (belly fat), supplementation with coconut oil (vs. soybean oil) showed an improvement in cholesterol profile and decreased waist circumference. Another study[52] found that MCT oil consumption led to a preferential loss in belly fat compared to corn oil consumption.

In other words, MCTs favor burning that stubborn belly fat.

Omega Fatty Acids: The Essential Fats for Weight Loss and Wellness

An important class of unsaturated fatty acids is the omega-3 and the omega-6 fatty acids. These fats are essential because they aren't made in the human body and need to be ingested in our diet. These fatty acids are 20 carbon-carbon chain long and are the building blocks of super-hormones known as eicosanoids. For a more detailed discussion of these fats, please refer to Appendix D.

Several studies have shown the beneficial effects omega-3 fats have on heart health and other chronic diseases, but a few recent ones have also shown their benefit in weight loss by increasing insulin sensitivity and warding off inflammation in fat cells[53].

Protein and Fat Lower Glycemic Index of Meal

Protein helps us lose weight by increasing the thermic loss of food, and fat promotes satiety so we are less likely to overeat. But the other valuable benefit of replacing carbohydrate calories with fat and protein is that they slow digestion and glucose uptake in the blood. This essentially lowers the GI of your food. For example, the GI of a pure mashed potato meal is 108, while the GI of the same meal with added fat (rapeseed oil) and protein (chicken breast) is only 54[54]. This has the effect of lowering your insulin (and leptin) levels. This reduces insulin-driven weight gain and helps re-sensitize your brain to leptin's signals. You feel full earlier and your metabolism is boosted. A double whammy for weight loss!

Fiber—The Satiety Carbohydrate

Fiber is technically a carbohydrate that adds no caloric value to food. It's found in the cells walls of wholesome sources of plant food. Fruits, vegetables, whole grains, lentils, legumes, and nuts are rich in fiber. Fiber helps weight loss in two ways. First, it slows the absorption of food in the stomach and regulates bowel movement. This prevents weight gain by slowing the rate at which glucose gets absorbed. The slow absorption of food keeps us feeling full longer. Again, this is akin to lowering the GI of food. This prevents us from getting hungry often and lowers total calorie intake by preventing overeating.

The second way it helps weight loss is via the action of colonic bacteria. Fermentation of fiber in the large intestines produces certain short chain fatty acids (SCFA) that are the preferred form of fuel for the probiotic bacteria in colon. This ensures colon health and protection from harmful pathogens and toxin producing bacterial[55]. This also helps prevent colon cancer[56]. Together, fiber and probiotic bacteria play a vital role in maintaining a healthy weight by regulating food absorption in the gut and by promoting colon health[57]. Probiotic bacteria found in fermented products like yogurt, kimchee, and sauerkraut also help with gut and colon health.

Modern factory-produced food is processed to remove fiber to improve texture. As a result, most packaged food is low in fiber and contributes to the growing rate of obesity. Examples are refined flour used in breads, cookies, and other baked foods.

By eating wholesome natural carbohydrates, you can ensure a good supply of fiber in the diet. The other advantage is that these wholesome carbohydrates are also rich in crucial vitamins, minerals, and antioxidants that support overall health and wellness.

Antioxidants: Burn Fat and Prevent Aging

Antioxidants play a vital role in prevention of chronic disease and aging (more in Appendix G). Recent studies have also shown beneficial effects on weight management.

The phenomenon of aging happens when cells in our bodies die, either naturally or from the effects of toxins in our diet and environment. Another cause for aging is when our cells stop performing the way they were meant to. An example of this is the function of collagen in our skin and other connective tissues. With age, the collagen in our body loses its elasticity, causing the formation of wrinkles.

Environmental and dietary toxins play a vital role in the aging phenomenon by generating free radicals and oxidation byproducts in our body that attack other healthy cells and reduce their functionality. Antioxidants, as the name suggests, are molecules that neutralize these harmful free radicals and protect our bodies from the ravages of aging. In addition to our body's own antioxidant defenses, the four most powerful antioxidants that should be included in our diets are: vitamins A, C, E, and selenium.

Apart from preventing premature aging, several studies have shown the benefits of antioxidants in enhancing weight loss. In one such study, it was found that foods high in antioxidants reduced belly fat and serum lipids (cholesterol and triglycerides) and lowered blood sugar[58].

Another study done on healthy young adults found that increasing dietary antioxidant content lowered blood pressure, blood sugar, and body mass index (an obesity metric)[59]. In another study done on 61 healthy young adults (ages 18-22), increasing vitamin A intake reduced belly fat[60].

In yet another study, 205 individuals were divided into three groups. One group consumed less than 2.5 servings of fruits and vegetables. The second group consumed between 2.5-5 servings of fruits and vegetables, and the third group consumed more than five servings of fruits and vegetables. The group that ate the most fruits and vegetables had the lowest waist circumference (belly fat)[61].

An Italian study done on adults between the ages of 18-66 found that taking 800-1000mg of antioxidants from fruits and vegetables had a significant improvement in how the body metabolizes carbohydrates and reduces weight gain. It's clear from these studies that eating antioxidants has a positive effect on weight reduction.

Dairy: It Does a Body Good

One often overlooked ingredient that is important for weight loss and greater fat oxidation (burning) is calcium. And dairy is a particularly rich source of it. Calcium has shown to promote fat breakdown and prevent fat storage.

Calcium has other benefits, like preventing bone loss (osteoporosis), regulation of blood pressure, and regularizing muscle contractions. It has also shown a preventive effect on breast and colon cancer.

In the Coronary Artery Risk Development in Young Adults (CARDIA) study[62], consisting of 3,157 adults between the ages of 18-30 years, researchers found that increased dairy consumption reduced weight gain and decreased the likelihood of developing type II diabetes and cardiovascular disease.

In another large study[63] with over 7,000 people ranging from 19-64 years of age, it was found that high consumption of dairy products was associated with a lower prevalence of obesity.

Apart from calcium, dairy is also a rich source of beneficial fats (conjugated linoleic acid, MUFA, and omega-3 fats), protein, and vitamin D, all of which have shown to contribute to weight loss and other health benefits. So dairy has an important place in your weight loss arsenal. If you are lactose intolerant, then consuming fermented dairy products like aged cheese and yogurt or even lactose-free milk will be beneficial. If you are a vegan, then try getting the RDA dosage of calcium via one of the many cruciferous vegetables or via supplementation.

Green Tea: The beverage of choice

Green tea (and to some extent, black tea) is also loaded with antioxidant polyphenols known as catechins. These catechins have shown benefit in preliminary clinical trials for lowering the risk of breast, prostate, ovarian, and endometrial cancers [64] and have shown to aid a reduction of LDL cholesterol and total cholesterol levels[65]. Green tea has also shown moderate thermic and fat-burning effects[66]. Even though there may be a slight weight loss advantage for people consuming green tea, I would advise against consuming it four hours before bedtime because it could interfere with normal sleep patterns, as green tea is also high in caffeine. This would in turn throw our leptin system off-balance. Green tea has also shown to be beneficial in the prevention of metabolic syndrome in a limited number of human trials[67]. This would imply beneficial effect on insulin sensitivity and weight loss.

Chapter 7

Five Keys to Successful Weight Loss

"Most weight loss diets center around portion control, which is just trying to eat smaller amounts of the same addictive foods. This approach inevitably fails."

Joel Fuhrman

In this chapter, you will learn:

- Practical tips necessary to lose weight and achieve wellness

It's time to take all this theory and apply it in easy-to-follow steps. Implementing these easy changes to your diet and exercise routine will not only cause effortless weight loss but will also keep your weight down in the long run. You won't feel deprived and lazy, but instead, you'll feel energetic and lively. In one word, following the suggestions in this section will help you *thrive!*

From what we have learned so far, weight loss can come naturally if we normalize the hormones that regulate our weight. Years of eating the wrong kinds of food due to rampant misinformation has caused the balance of these hormones to shift us in the direction of obesity. The goal of any weight-loss program should be to address these underlying hormonal causes. Without addressing these causes, any diet or exercise program is destined to fail. Here are the main goals that need to be addressed:

1) **Lower insulin levels:** Consume meals consisting mostly of protein and fat and/or always combine wholesome carbohydrates with proteins and fats. Lowered insulin levels directly increase fat burning and prevent fat accumulation.

2) **Increase leptin sensitivity:** By lowering our insulin levels (goal 1), you will also lower your leptin levels. This will sensitize your brain to leptin's signals. Once you achieve leptin sensitivity, your brain will listen to leptin's "stop eating" signal and keep hunger at bay and ramp up your metabolism for increased fat burning.

3) **Use the thermic advantage of food:** Eat foods that are high in protein to increase thermic loss. This boosts metabolism and cuts the amount of available calories for weight gain, since some of the calories are lost in the process of digestion. It's like cutting calories without cutting calories.

4) **Eat foods that satisfy your brain:** A satisfied brain is the key to having a fast metabolism. Eating healthy fats along with protein and fiber-rich foods slow digestion and the absorption of glucose in the blood. This effectively lowers the glycemic index of the meal, which prevents insulin spiking. This prevents hunger pangs and keeps the brain satisfied.

5) **Manage stress:** Lower cortisol levels through moderate exercise, yoga, tai chi, and other breathing/meditation techniques. High cortisol levels are a big contributor to belly fat, which is one of the biggest reasons for most chronic diseases.

Keeping these goals in mind, I have designed the 5 Golden Rules of weight loss:

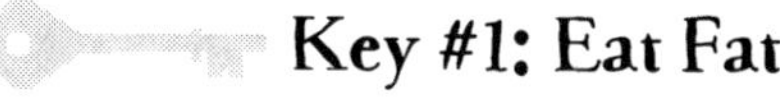 Key #1: Eat Fat

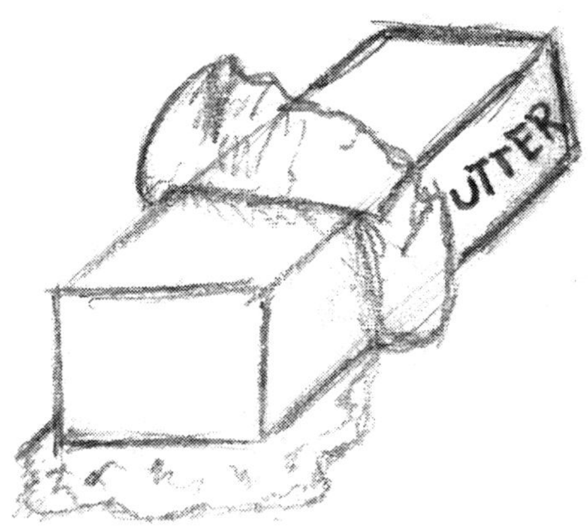

Fat is your friend. Even though fat has twice the number of calories as protein or carbohydrates, it contributes to the satiety factor of food. Fat slows down sugar uptake in blood, lowering your insulin levels. This minimizes insulin-driven weight gain. It keeps you satisfied and prevents you from overeating. Incorporating healthy fats from nuts, avocados, olives, butter, and coconuts in your diet will reduce your overall calorie consumption. Fat is also the building block of all the hormones, so it contributes to healthy levels of hormones that regulate body weight. For more information on fat, see Appendix D.

Fat slows down sugar uptake in blood, lowering your insulin levels.

Having Medium Chain Triglycerides (MCT) from coconut oil and butter gives your body an easy source of energy and teaches your body to burn stored body fat. Consuming Mono Unsaturated Fatty Acids (MUFA) from nuts and olive oil targets belly fat and confers heart health. Fats from grass-fed dairy have the ideal omega-6/omega-3 ratio of 1 to 4. This helps lower systemic inflammation, the main driver for all chronic disease. Additionally, fats from butter and clarified butter give you radiant skin, luxurious hair, and healthy nails. In one sentence, "fat will help you lose fat and make you beautiful."

Must-eat fats:

Nut butters (almonds, walnuts, pecans, macadamia, cashew, pistachio) are a rich source of MUFA that help target belly fat. Coconut oil and cream of coconut are rich in antifungal and antimicrobial components and also MCTs. Red palm kernel oil is also a rich source of antioxidants and vitamin E ; it's also a rich source of MCTs. Dark chocolate (80% or more) is also a good source of MUFA and antioxidants, so eat it in moderation (only because of the sugar content in chocolate). Also don't forget to enjoy that utterly buttery delicious butter from grass-fed cows!

Fats to Avoid

All Trans-fats. Most refined vegetable oils (canola, sunflower, and rapeseed) are refined at high temperatures and treated with chemicals, so you should avoid them. These vegetable fats are a rich source of omega-6 fatty acids, which are highly pro-inflammatory. Unless the vegetable oil consumption is balanced with omega-3 fats from grass-fed dairy and fish oils, it will increase systemic inflammation.

Suggested use:

Fat is best used raw as salad dressings and seasoning. Extra virgin unrefined oil (olive, avocado, hemp, walnut, flax) are a rich source of antioxidants and heating them to high temperatures destroys these antioxidants. So using them raw as dips or dressings is the best way to eat them. Other healthy fats in nut butters (almond, walnut, peanut) are best used as salad dips and spreads. The best fats for cooking are refined avocado, clarified butter, and coconut oil, as they have a high smoke point. The smoke point of oil is when it visibly starts smoking. This disintegrates the fats into dangerous free radicals.

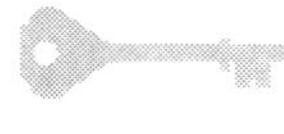

Key #2: Have a protein-rich meal within an hour of waking up

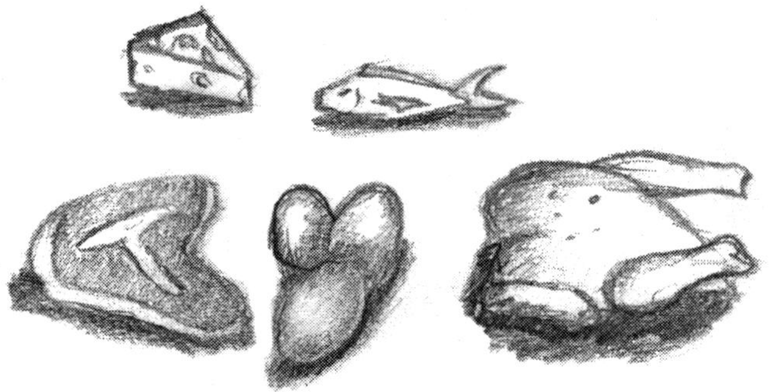

Protein boosts the thermic effect of food and helps kick-start your metabolism into high gear so you burn extra calories during the day. Add a dose of healthy fats to this and some fiber-rich carbohydrates to keep you satisfied and prevent overeating throughout the day. Eat between-meal snacks that are rich in fat and protein (such as nuts) to normalize insulin levels and prevent hunger pangs.

Must-have proteins:

Deep-sea cold-water fish. Free pastured poultry, eggs, dairy, and meats. Avocados, hemp, chia and flax seeds (also a good source of omega-3 fats), walnuts, pecans, pistachios, and macadamia. Lentils and legumes (mix a few different kinds to have the complete amino acid profile). A whey protein shake is a good option for a quick protein snack. For vegetarians, there are excellent sources of proteins that are also rich in healthy fats. Please refer to Appendix B, for a list of healthy vegetarian proteins.

Protein boosts the thermic effect of food and helps kick-start your metabolism

Proteins to Avoid:

Factory-processed meats (sausages, pepperoni, bacon, etc.). Wheat gluten and soy isolates, mainly because almost all wheat and soy protein are derived from genetically modified grains.

Key #3: Eat Healthy Carbohydrates

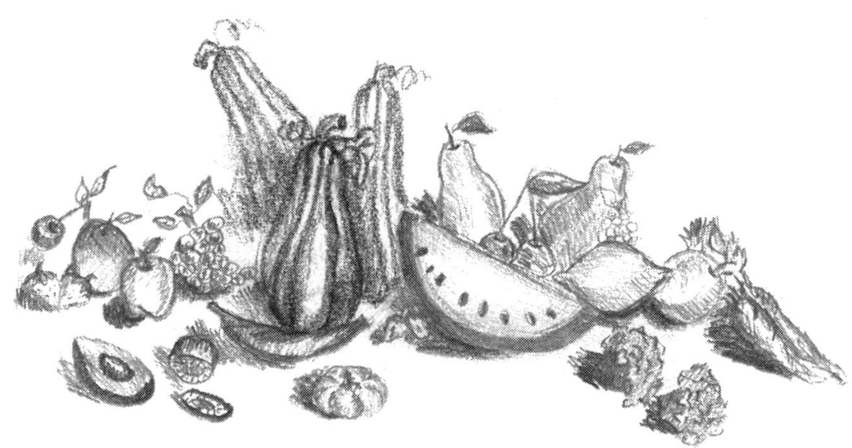

Carbohydrates are a rich source of fiber and antioxidants. Have plenty of green vegetables (leafy and cruciferous), nuts, berries, spices, and herbs to boost thermic activity and to get a healthy dose of antioxidants and fiber. Legumes and nuts are also a rich source of thermic protein, fiber, and antioxidants, all of which make for a good fat-burning diet.

Must-have carbohydrates:

Leafy greens: spinach, kale, collard greens. Cruciferous vegetables like cauliflower, broccoli, cabbage, bok choy, watercress, lettuce. Fruits like apples, pears, kiwi, avocado and all berries (strawberry, blackberry, blueberry, raspberry). Pulses like lentils, beans, and legumes. Herbs like cilantro, parsley, basil, sage, oregano, ginger, and garlic; and spices like turmeric, cloves, cayenne pepper, black pepper etc. All nuts.

Carbohydrates to Avoid:

Easily digested carbohydrates like rice, wheat, sugars, potatoes, and other starchy vegetables. All processed carbohydrates like cookies, Twinkies, donuts, pastries, cakes, etc. All sugary beverages including fruit juices, which are nothing more than concentrated fructose (a cousin of sucrose or table sugar).

Key #4: Manage Stress

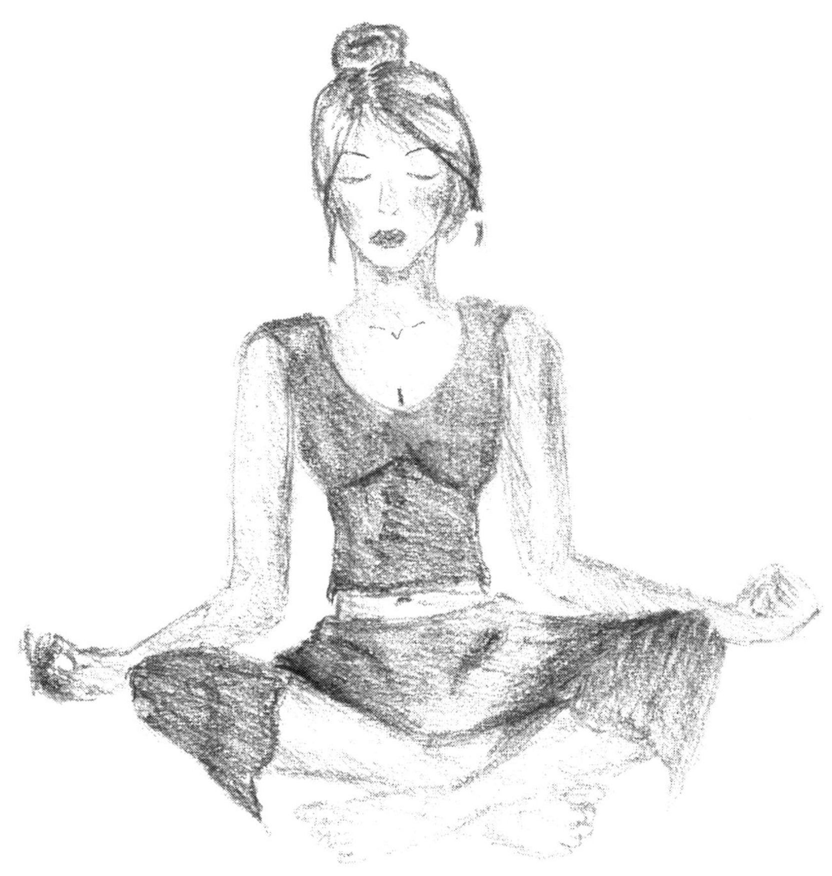

Stress is one of the key reasons for impaired insulin and leptin response because of high levels of circulating blood sugar (due to cortisol). Manage stress with breathing techniques, yoga, pranayama, tai chi, and other relaxation techniques. Watch a comedy movie every once in a while, and maintain a generally positive outlook on life.

Manage stress with breathing techniques, yoga, pranayama, tai chi, and other relaxation techniques.

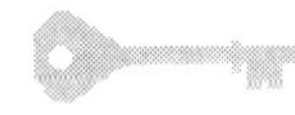

Key #5: Cheat once in a while

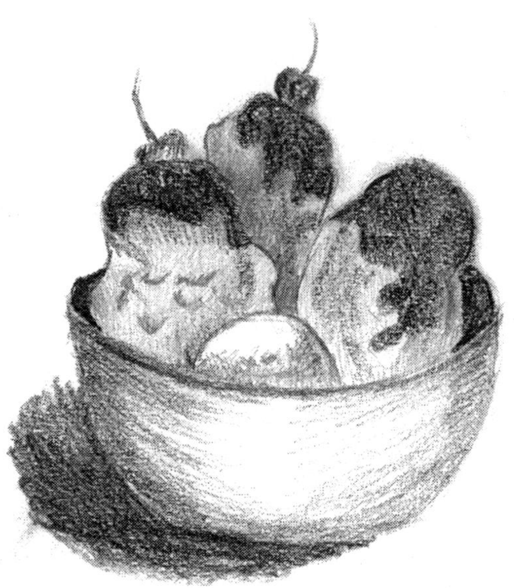

Initially, it's important to eat foods that reduce our leptin levels so that our brain gets sensitized to leptin's signals. Once our brain is sensitized to leptin, we need an occasional leptin boost for the brain to keep suppressing hunger and boosting our metabolic rate. This is when a cheat meal helps, and here's how:

Since leptin is produced in the fat cells of our body, there will be a drop in leptin levels as we lose body fat. This will cause an increase in hunger and a suppression of metabolic rate. This is counterproductive to weight loss. This is homeostasis at work trying to maintain your body weight set-point. Eventually, you will reach the point of marginal returns where your weight loss will reduce to a crawl and you will experience unabated hunger pangs. At this point, it is helpful to boost your leptin levels by boosting your insulin levels.

Once in ten days or so, you MUST indulge in one cheat meal

A cheat meal is nothing but a meal consisting of easily digested carbohydrates (high Glycemic Index). This boosts your insulin levels in the short term and as a result, your leptin levels as well. Once in ten days or so, you MUST indulge in one cheat meal consisting of high-GI carbohydrates like pizza, pastries, cookies and ice cream. This will quickly boost insulin and leptin levels. Once the leptin levels go up, the brain suppresses hunger and keeps your metabolism revved up.

A cheat meal is fun and helps you break through any weight loss plateaus that will eventually happen. Having the occasional treat also prevents psychological burnout and ensures the long-term success of sticking to your diet. As you lose more and more body fat, you will have to increase the frequency of cheat meals. Once you are below 10% body fat level (six-pack begins to show), you will have to indulge in a cheat meal once about every 3-4 days.

Chapter 8

The 5 Common Pitfalls to Avoid

"Good things do not come easy. The road is lined with pitfalls."

Desi Arnaz

In this chapter, you will learn:

- Some of the things that will seem like the logical thing to do in your weight loss journey but are pitfalls in disguise.

Here are some of the common pitfalls to avoid in your weight-loss journey.

The reason I call them pitfalls is because on the surface, they seem to be the right thing to do, but looking closely, you will realize how they could jeopardize your weight-loss goals.

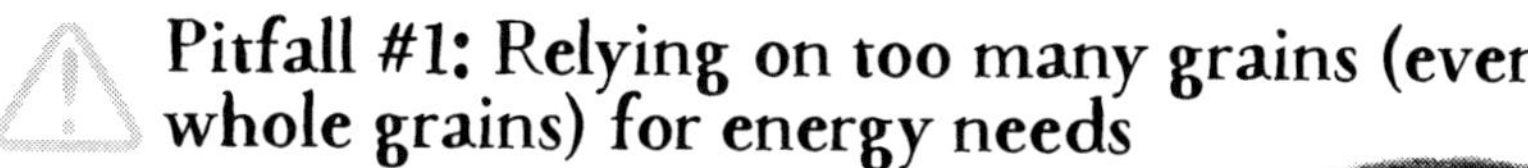

Pitfall #1: Relying on too many grains (even whole grains) for energy needs

Grains are a good source of certain essential vitamins, minerals, and fiber. However, they are also a rich source of easily digested carbohydrates. Wheat is the most widely consumed grain, and a majority of the carbohydrate in wheat is in the form of amylopectin, which is an easily digested form of carbohydrate. Dr.

William Davis, the author of The New York Times bestseller *Wheat Belly*, calls wheat a super carbohydrate because of its amylopectin content. According to him, wheat ramps up hunger and is highly addictive. The GI of wheat bread is 69, which is higher than that of table sugar (59)[68]. Refined wheat flour, found in most bakery goodies, has a GI of 100, which is equivalent to glucose. So eating whole wheat bread is worse than eating sugar in terms of insulin response (and the resultant weight gain). Most other grains are also a rich source of carbohydrates, making them prime candidates for weight gain. So have grains in moderation.

It's best to have your carbohydrates from vegetables, as they are low in carbohydrates and higher in antioxidants, fiber, and other nutritional components.

It's best to have your carbohydrates from vegetables, as they are low in carbohydrates and higher in antioxidants, fiber, and other nutritional components. Berries are also a good source of low-GI carbohydrates. So are nuts, lentils, and legumes. Sprouted lentils like mung beans make a nutritious low-GI snack.

Of notable mention is quinoa, marketed as a grain but technically a nut from the Amaranthaceae family. It has the complete amino acid profile, so makes for an excellent source of protein as well.

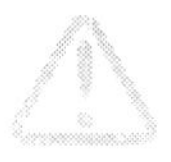

Pitfall #2: Over-exercising

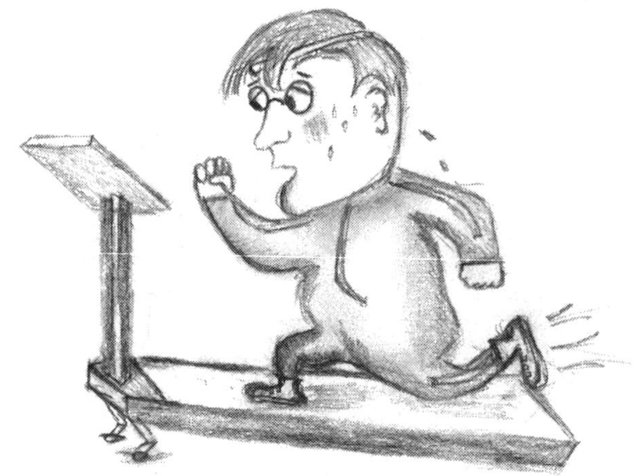

As mentioned in Chapter 5, exercise will cause an increase in appetite. The more you exercise, the more you will have to exert willpower in order to stop yourself from eating. Furthermore, exercise is a kind of stress, albeit of a controlled variety. It does make the body stronger and resilient and has a host of other benefits, but when it comes to exercise, there is such a thing as too much of a good thing. Avoid long duration cardio, because it induces a prolonged stress response. It's best to exercise moderately. If you love going to the gym, make sure you do no more than 45 minutes of exercise in any workout (2-3 times a week) and if you love cardio, then make sure you do no more than 30-45 minutes of moderate intensity (walking, light jogging, hiking) 2-3 times a week. Do yoga, pranayama, or tai chi, and play some sports. Above all, stay active and moving throughout the day.

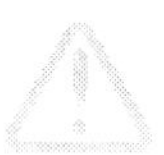

Pitfall #3: Eating Low-Fat

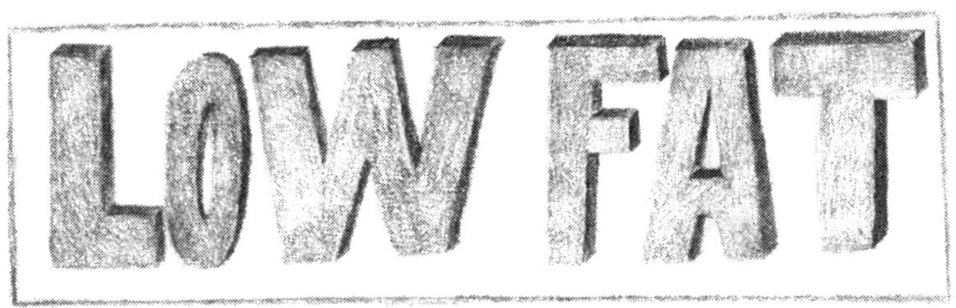

"Low-fat" was synonymous with "healthy" until a few years back (and even now, for many). Only as recently as in the last 8-10 years have the virtues of fat been discovered and how important it is for overall health and vitality. The weight loss benefits of fat came to the forefront with the popularity of low-carbohydrate diets. Fat being the cause for weight gain has been so ingrained in our minds that even now, you watch people at the grocery store and you will see them reach out for low-fat/skim milk instead of regular milk even though regular milk has a lower GI than skim milk (which has added sugar to compensate for some of the lost flavor from removing fat). Most people still go for the low-fat yogurt and low-fat ice cream when the real enemy is the sugar in these low-fat processed foods. Every time someone sees me eating a handful of walnuts in the afternoon, they ask, "Aren't you afraid of gaining weight?"

> The worst thing you can do in your quest to lose weight is to avoid fat.

The worst thing you can do in your quest to lose weight is to avoid fat. When you avoid fat, you compensate for that with calories from carbohydrates, since most natural sources of protein are also high in fat. What ends up happening is insulin-driven weight gain.

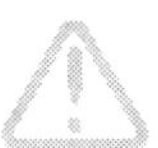

Pitfall #4: Eating Too Many Fruits

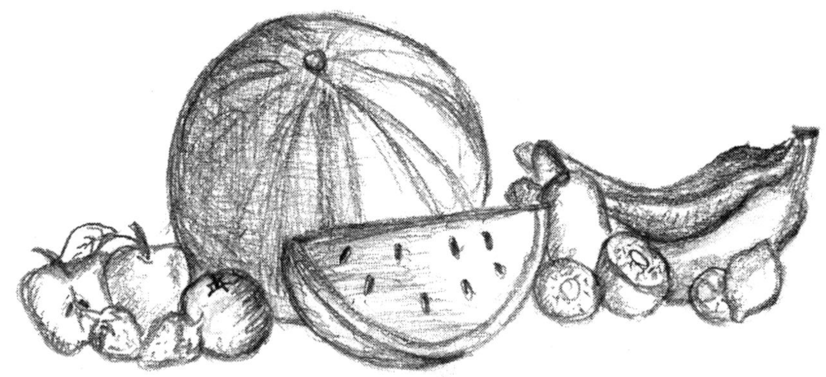

The primary form of sugar in fruits is fructose, which is a close cousin of sucrose (table sugar). Fructose has shown to have a lower Glycemic Index so it is often thought of as being healthier. Fructose is not broken down in the gut (hence the lower GI) but almost entirely processed in the liver. Overdoing fruits, especially in juice form, overburdens the liver and contributes to fatty liver disease. It has also shown to be a bigger contributor to aging from Advanced Glycation End-products (AGE) (more on this in Appendix F).

Since fructose doesn't immediately raise blood glucose levels it also doesn't raise insulin and leptin levels. By circumventing the usual digestive channel, fructose, has little effect on hunger (since leptin levels don't rise) and the person continues to eat. Due to this fructose, when taken in large quantities, has shown to induce leptin resistance in animal models. So stick to the low-fructose varieties of fruits like apples, peaches, apricots, berries (all varieties), plums, and grapefruit. Eat mangoes, pineapple, papaya, and melons in moderation. And also if possible only eat whole fruit. The fiber content in fruit balances out the fructose and slows down its absorption, keeping the liver happy and healthy. Remember, never drink your fruit and always eat it.

fructose, when taken in large quantities, has shown to induce leptin resistance

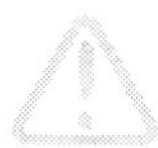

Pitfall #5: Drinking Diet Soda

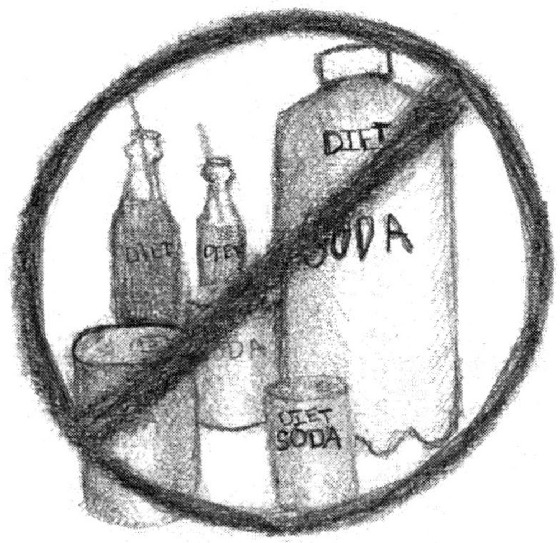

Until recently, diet soda was thought of as a better alternative to regular soda for people wanting to lose weight. And who is to blame for that? If something can taste as sweet as the real thing and yet have no calories, it's a Godsend. But recent research has shown that people who drink diet soda are more likely to overeat and end up consuming more calories compared to regular soda drinkers. Additionally, diet soda has shown to cause insulin and leptin resistance.

In a nine-year follow-up study, diet soda consumption showed increased waist circumference compared to non-drinkers[69]. Another study, including 2,371 girls between the ages of 9-19 years, has shown that the consumption of both diet and regular soda led to an increase in total daily calorie intake[70].

A possible mechanism proposed for diet soda related weight gain is something like this: the brain senses the sweet taste and expects a quick surge of glucose. It commands the pancreas to start producing insulin in anticipation of incoming sugar. But when the glucose doesn't arrive, the brain ramps up hunger. This delivers a double whammy by putting your body in storage mode and making you hungry. The leptin increase that follows the insulin rise contributes to aggravating the leptin resistance. This could explain the increased hunger as a result of diet soda consumption.

> Essentially diet soda delivers a double whammy.

Also, the sweet taste minus the calories increases the cravings for easy carbohydrates. Again, the increase in the consumption of easy carbohydrates as a result of cravings will lead to leptin resistance. A deadly catch 22 situation!

Essentially diet soda delivers a double whammy. Increased leptin resistance sends the brain a "starvation" signal and increased insulin production puts your body in storage mode. You can see how diet soda doesn't stand up to its claims of being diet friendly.

Chapter 9

A Food Pyramid for Weight Loss and Wellness

"He who distinguishes the true savor of his food can never be a glutton; he who does not cannot be otherwise."

Henry David Thoreau

In this chapter, you will learn:

- What a wellness food pyramid should be, based on the science of nutrition.
- How you can incorporate the simple rules of nutrition and lifestyle in this easy to follow pyramid.

In Part 1, we learned how excess insulin from overindulgence in carbohydrates makes us fat by switching our body into fat-storage mode. Furthermore, we saw how this pattern of eating causes leptin resistance, which moves our weight set-point toward preferential weight gain. The resulting weight gain comes with its own suite of metabolic disorders that are at the root of today's modern degenerative diseases.

In Part 2, we learned practical tips on how to reverse these hormonal abnormalities to get lean and achieve a better state of wellness.

In this chapter, I condense everything and put it into an easy-to-follow food pyramid. Eat according to this pyramid and your weight-loss journey will be easy. At the same time, you will improve your overall wellness and prevent premature aging. I call it the AXIOM™ pyramid and here's why:

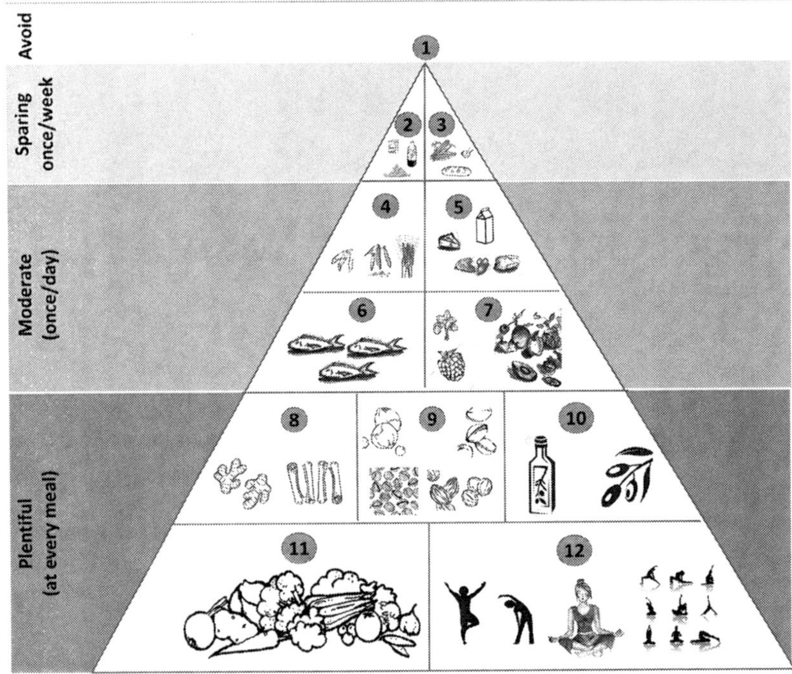

Legend:

1. Trans Fats and Processed Meats	2. Sugars, Syrups, Jams, Sugary Cereals, Soda
3. White Rice, Starchy Vegetables, Refined Wheat Flour, White Bread, Corn	4. Whole Grains: Lentils, Beans and Legumes
5. Free Pastured Butter, Eggs, Poultry, Red-meat, Dairy, Coconut oil, Dark Chocolate	6. Fatty Deep Sea Fish
7. Berries and Low Carbohydrate Fruits	8. Herbs and Spices
9. Nuts and Seeds	10. Olive, Flax Seed, Avocado, and Hemp Oil
11. Non-starchy Vegetables	12. Yoga, Tai Chi, Moderate Exercise and Meditation (daily)

Figure 15: The AXIOM Pyramid.

The AXIOM™ Pyramid

The AXIOM™ pyramid is based on three guiding principles of wellness:

- **A**ntio**X**idants for protecting us from premature aging and improving overall wellness.
- **I**nsulin management for weight regulation and overall wellness.
- Balancing the intake of **OM**ega fats for preventing chronic disease.

Implementing the AXIOM™ principle in our daily life will not only make us lean but also give us freedom from most modern degenerative diseases like heart disease, diabetes, certain cancers, auto-immune disorders, age-related dementia, and premature aging.

AXIOM™ principle in our daily life will not only make us lean but also give us freedom from most modern degenerative diseases

The AXIOM™ pyramid in Figure 15 is similar to the USDA food pyramid. You eat more of the foods at the bottom of the pyramid and eat less of the foods on top. The types of foods are divided into three shaded regions.

Let's go down through the pyramid, starting from the top, and lay down the ground rules of using it:

The 'Avoid' list

On the apex of the pyramid is the *Avoid list*: all Trans-fats and hydrogenated fats. Read labels carefully; manufacturers label their products as 'zero Trans-fats' when they have partially hydrogenated fat which is another name for 'Trans-fats.' The FDA allows manufacturers to label anything containing less than 0.5g /serving of Trans-fat as "zero" Trans-fat. If you are consuming multiple servings of such a food, then the total amount of Trans-fats will add up. Remember, there is no safe level of Trans-fats for human consumption. Always read labels before buying a product (even the so-called health bars) and if it says it has partially hydrogenated fats, put it back on the shelf. Vegetable shortenings like Crisco™ are also Trans-fat that are used as a replacement for butter in many baked confections.

Also to avoid are all processed meats like bacon, sausages, pepperoni, bologna and other deli meats as they are mostly made from factory produced meat and pumped with preservatives and other chemicals to prolong shelf life and enhance flavor.

The Eat Sparingly list:

The *Eat Sparingly list* is the sweet and refined processed carbohydrate category: all items with sugar and high-fructose corn syrup, like soft drinks, candy, and sugary cereals (corn flakes, Cheerios®, and most kids' cereals). It also includes refined processed carbohydrates such as white bread, pasta, bakery items (cakes, pastries, donuts, etc.), white rice, corn products, potato products (chips, fries, etc.), and refined flour items (Indian naan, donuts, pizza, etc.). Eat only once a week at most (or at cheat meals).

The Eat Moderately list:

The *Eat Moderately* section of the pyramid has four subsections. One of them contains whole grains, legumes, pulses, beans, and lentils. These foods provide fiber along with essential vitamins and minerals. They are also rich in certain essential amino acids, so vegetarians should mix several of them in a meal to ensure they get the full spectrum of essential amino acids for protein synthesis. They also have a lower GI so they help manage insulin levels during the day. Have once a day.

The second section has wholesome fats from butter, clarified butter, red palm oil, and coconut oil. These fats are rich in certain vitamins and antioxidants and are less prone to turning rancid. They also have fats that are good for gut health and for their antimicrobial and antiviral properties. The shorter-chain fatty acids present in coconut oil are readily burned for energy. Clarified butter can be used for any frying or deep-frying and is preferable to vegetable oils that are more delicate at high heats, and turn rancid more quickly. This section also contains *Poultry and Dairy* foods. These are high in protein as well as essential vitamins and minerals. Eating some of the fermented items from this section like yogurt, buttermilk, and cheese will help restore probiotic balance in the colon for better digestive health. These foods will also provide some of the daily fat needs. The lacto-ovo vegetarians can stick to eggs and dairy, and the meat eaters can have poultry as well. You can eat 1-2 whole eggs daily, but discarding the yolk is throwing away the most nutritious part of the egg. Eat them whole! Overall, you can have 2-3 servings daily from this group, either in one meal or spread over 2-3 meals.

The third section contains deep-sea cold water fish that are a good source of essential omega-3 fats.

The fourth section contains berries and other low-carbohydrate fruits. These are a good source of antioxidants that prevent many chronic diseases and also prevent premature aging.

The Eat Plentiful list:

The *Eat Plentiful list* is divided into two layers.

The first layer has all the sources of healthy fats like fish and krill oils for essential omega-3 fats; nuts for mono-unsaturated fatty acids (MUFA); and other plant oils that are rich in the parent form of omega-3 fats like olive, avocado, flax and hemp seed oils. It also has herbs and spices that are antioxidant powerhouses.

The next layer has all the vegetables from the cruciferous family and all the other greens and many other vegetables that are rich in plant polyphenols, antioxidants, vitamins, and minerals. These foods must be had at every meal.

In the second layer, I added another category for moderate exercise, yoga, tai chi, Pilates, meditation, and other stress relaxation activities, and they should be a part of daily life.

Follow this pyramid as a general guideline to decide how much of each kind of food you should eat. Make sure you buy locally farmed organic produce and free pasture meats, dairy, poultry and eggs. Seafood should be cold water wild caught and not farmed. Avoid the typical supermarket processed fare. Eating in accordance with this pyramid should help you get rid of any hunger pangs and cravings and should help you achieve a higher level of wellness and vitality. Weight loss will be a pleasant side effect.

buy locally farmed organic produce and free pasture meats, dairy, poultry and eggs

Epilogue

Our diets in the last half-century have been shaped by pseudoscience and rampant misinformation driven by food politics and corporate bottom lines. The resulting nutritional disaster has not only made us fatter and sicker but also literally made us prisoners of our own bodies. We try to break free every now and then, but end up in the same (body) prison, which only gets bigger every time we come back.

The real cause of weight gain is our bodies' altered hormonal state brought on by the modern Western processed diet. This altered hormonal state is causing our bodies to be in constant fat storage mode. Everything we eat, the body wants to store as fat. The result: excessive hunger and lethargy! This has slowly pushed our bodyweight set-point toward increasing adiposity.

In this state, when we try to lose weight by eating less and exercising more, powerful evolutionary forces of HUNGER and METABOLISM come into play to maintain our bodyweight set-point. The "*eat less and exercise more*" prescription merely addresses the symptom of weight gain without fixing the real underlying cause. This is why we can't achieve long-term weight loss and we keep coming back to our natural bodyweight set-point. Nature cannot be defeated!

My hope is that after reading this book, you realize that in order to achieve lasting weight loss, we need to address the real hormonal cause of weight gain, so we can naturally move our bodyweight set-point toward leanness. When we do this, the same evolutionary forces that now prevent us from losing weight will help us lose weight effortlessly.

Work *with* nature, not *against* it!

"Treat the cause, not the effect."

– Dr. Edward Bach

7 Day Meal Plan

10 simple commonsense rules to follow:

1) Eat deliberately and consciously. This means you savor every bite and never eat in a hurry, because it takes about 15-20 minutes for the leptin levels to rise and for the brain to sense the leptin signals. Stop when full. This means no watching TV and stuffing yourself. No need to count calories.

2) Drink plenty of water and stay hydrated.

3) You can have three main meals. The mid-meal snacks are not mandatory; have them only if you get hungry between meals. Once your body is adapted to burning stored body fat, it will easily switch over to burning stored body fat for energy between meals, so hunger won't be an issue between meals. It is okay to skip meals if you are not hungry.

4) If in stress and reaching for food, ask yourself if you are really hungry or if you just want to escape the feeling of stress and anxiety.

5) Dinner should be three hours before bedtime. If hungry at bedtime, have a handful of nuts or a cheese stick or some other low-carbohydrate snack.

6) Don't overcook fat. Cook in avocado oil, clarified butter, or coconut oil. Canola and safflower oils are okay in moderation. Avoid deep-frying, but if you do, do it in clarified butter or avocado oil. Don't fear butter!

7) Use herbs and spices (not salt) liberally.

8) Be imaginative and experiment with food. As long as you are eating the right ingredients, feel free to mix and match according to personal taste.

9) Always prefer locally produced and farmed organic produce and free pasture meats/eggs/dairy. Avoid the typical supermarket processed fare.

10) Above all, enjoy what you eat!

Day 1:

Breakfast

Stir-fry quinoa in butter with vegetables (carrots, zucchini, cabbage, Brussels sprouts, etc.) topped with cilantro. Salt and spices added to taste.

Mid-morning Snack (optional)

Handful of almonds or walnuts.

Lunch

Lentil soup with vegetables and beans. Eat with steamed quinoa or pearled barley.

Mid afternoon Snack (optional)

Celery with almond or walnut butter.

Dinner

Chickpea salad with tomatoes, grated cheese, avocados, hard-boiled eggs, spinach or kale. Topped with flaxseed, hemp, or extra virgin olive oil.

Day 2:

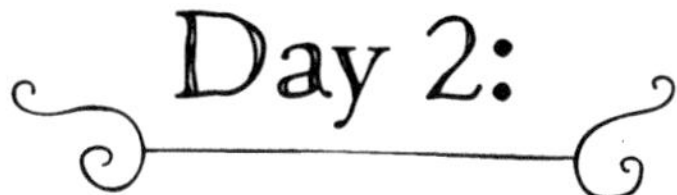

Breakfast

2-3 egg with cheese omelet with bell peppers, onions, mushrooms, spinach, kale, etc. Salt/pepper to taste. Cooked in grass-fed butter. Unsweetened coffee/tea or tomato juice.

Mid-morning Snack (optional)

One apple

Lunch

Mung bean noodles with vegetables and organic non-GMO tofu. Spices and salt added to taste.

Mid-afternoon Snack (optional)

Carrots or celery sticks with hummus.

Dinner

Mung bean-batter pancakes (chilla) prepared in butter with mint, cilantro, and ground peanut chutney.

Day 3:

Breakfast

Steamed quinoa topped with clarified butter, shredded coconut, and peanut/cilantro chutney with unsweetened coffee/tea or tomato juice. Few cottage cheese cubes (paneer).

Mid-morning Snack (optional)

Handful of walnuts.

Lunch

Chili paneer (cottage cheese) with sweet peppers and steamed quinoa.

Mid-afternoon Snack (optional)

Pearled barley toast with pesto sauce.

Dinner

Baked zucchini boats stuffed with ricotta cheese and fresh tomato sauce topped with mozzarella cheese. Sprinkle with chopped fresh basil/parsley.

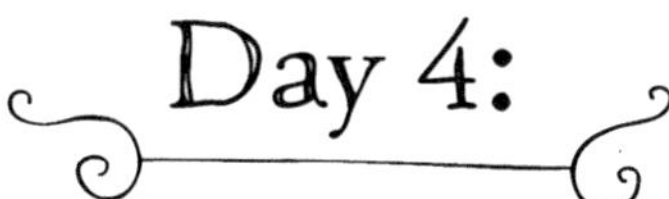

Breakfast

Egg salad made with 2-3 boiled eggs, one tablespoon organic mayo or hummus, grated celery, one teaspoon grass-fed butter, salt and black pepper to taste. Unsweetened tea/coffee or tomato juice.

Mid-morning Snack (optional)

Two teaspoons peanut or almond butter.

Lunch

Sautéed chicken breast with French beans, tomatoes, spinach, and kidney beans. Add salt, spices, and herbs to taste.

Mid-afternoon Snack (optional)

Cheese-stuffed baked jalapeno peppers.

Dinner

Stuffed avocado with tuna, tomatoes, onions, and cilantro. Salt and crushed pepper to taste.

Day 5:

Breakfast

Yams stuffed with ricotta cheese, mushrooms and Italian spices. Coffee or unsweetened tea.

Mid-morning Snack (optional)

Cheese sticks

Lunch

Antipasto salad with artichoke, olives, mushrooms, cabbage, and feta cheese. Ranch or bleu cheese dressing.

Mid-afternoon Snack (optional)

Handful of almonds or walnuts or pistachios.

Dinner

Chicken stew with squash, zucchini, carrots, and celery. Topped with sage, basil, and cilantro. Salt and pepper to taste.

Day 6:

Breakfast

3 pastured eggs scrambled in grass fed butter with mushrooms and celery. Salt pepper to taste. Unsweetened tea/coffee or tomato juice.

Mid-morning Snack (optional)

Two teaspoons peanut or almond butter.

Lunch

Butter chicken/lamb with one cup steamed quinoa.

Mid-afternoon Snack (optional)

Zucchini rolls with goat cheese and sun-dried tomatoes.

Dinner

Eggplant parmigiana (without pasta) with steamed vegetables.

Day 7:

Breakfast

Power Smoothie: blend coconut milk, berries, walnuts, kale, flax seeds, hemp seeds with water (for consistency) in a blender. Mix protein powder (optional).

Mid-morning Snack (optional)

Smoked salmon on barley crackers.

Lunch

Mung Bean noodles with veggies and chicken.

Mid-afternoon Snack (optional)

1oz. dark semisweet chocolate (80% or more cocoa)

Dinner

Steamed fish and chickpea salad with bell peppers, zucchini and tomatoes topped with spicy sauce and toasted sesame oil.

APPENDIXES

REFERENCE MATERIAL

Appendix A

Belly Fat Busting Superfoods

This section contains a list of all the flat belly superfoods that will help you attain your desired weight without starving you. Additionally these foods are a rich source of essential vitamins, minerals and antioxidants so they will help you achieve a higher level of wellness and vitality. Most of these foods are a must have in your pantry if you are serious about your health.

Nut-up to Cut-up

Nuts and seeds are rich in monounsaturated fatty acids (MUFA) and fiber, both of which are essential to losing belly fat. Nuts are also rich in thermogenic protein and also provide antioxidants that neutralize the oxidation from dietary toxins and environmental pollutants. This prevents premature aging.

Here is a list of all the nuts and seeds that belong in your pantry:

Almonds	Macadamia	Hemp
Walnuts	Brazil nuts	Sunflower
Pistachios	Cashews	Pumpkin
Peanuts	Pine nuts	Chia
Hazelnuts	Pecans	Flax

Go Green to Be Lean

Vegetables are a good source of healthy carbohydrates, antioxidants, important vitamins, and trace minerals. They also provide good amounts of fiber. They should be had at every meal. Here is a list of all the vegetables that you should be eating:

Kale	Carrots	Arugula
Spinach	Leeks	Asparagus
Cabbage	Bok Choy	Endive
Lettuce	Okra	Kohlrabi
Celery	Brussel Sprouts	Mustard Greens
Collard Greens	Beets	Pea Pods
Bell Peppers	Radishes	Turnip
Swiss chard	Eggplant	Watercress
Moringa Oliefera (Indian Drumsticks)	Zucchini	Yams
Butternut	Broccoli	Sugar Snap Peas
	Artichokes	

Eat Fat to Beat Fat

Fats improve palatability of food, satisfy the brain, slow the absorption of sugars, keep cells healthy, and build hormones.

Medium chain triglycerides (MCT) teach your body to burn stored body fat and monounsaturated fatty acids (MUFA) keep your heart healthy and burn belly fat. Fat is your biggest friend in your quest to lose fat. Here is a list of fats to include in your diet:

Cooking Medium:

Palm Oil	Avocado Oil	Butter
Olive Oil	Coconut Oil	Clarified Butter (Ghee)

Dips and Salads:

Almond Oil	Pecan Oil	Wheat Germ Oil
Macadamia Oil	Pine nut oil	Walnut oil
Brazil nut Oil	Pistachio Oil	Flax Seed oil
Cashew Oil	Hemp Seed oil	Acai Oil

Supplement:

Blackcurrant Seed oil	Borage Seed oil
Evening Primrose oil	Black seed oil

Berry to feel Merry (and other low-fructose fruits)

Berries and other fruits provide important vitamins and trace minerals. They also provide a good amount of antioxidants and healthy fiber. Although fructose, the sugar found in fruits, has a low glycemic index (meaning it spikes the blood sugar slowly), it causes a higher level of glycation of other fats and proteins in the body. This contributes to a greater production of AGE free radicals that contribute to accelerated aging. So have fruits in moderation and don't overdo the especially sweet ones (mangoes, pineapple, cantaloupes, grapes, and bananas). Overeating fruits has also shown to induce leptin resistance, which would be counterproductive to weight loss. Here is a list of fruits to have in your diet:

Blackberry	Guava	Kiwi
Blueberry	Apricot	Gooseberry (Amla)
Strawberry	cherries	Tomato
Raspberry	Apple	Olives
Pear	Olives	Papaya
Nectarine	Avocado	
Peach	Grapefruit	

Spice for Belly-fat Slice

Spices and herbs provide a concentrated source of antiaging antioxidants. They also help increase insulin sensitivity, so they help with weight loss. Spices like turmeric have also shown to be beneficial in the fight against cancer. Use spices liberally in everyday cooking. Here is the list for your pantry:

Turmeric	Bay Leaf	Lavender
Sumac	Borage	Mace
Ginger	Fenugreek	Marjoram
Cilantro	Cardamom	Nutmeg
Mint	Caper	Oregano
Parsley	Cinnamon	Peppermint
Basil	Clove	Rosemary
Sage	Cumin	Star Anise
Black pepper	Curry Leaves	Szechuan Pepper
White pepper	Dill	Thyme
Anise	Mustard	Terragon
Carom Seeds	Fennel	Willow Herb
Annatto	Garlic	White Mustard
Asfoetida	Horseradish	
Basil	Licorice	

Dairy for Skin Like A Fairy

Dairy is a good source of calcium, magnesium, and other important minerals. Free pasture (or grass fed) dairy also has the ideal omega-6/3 fatty acid ratio for chronic disease prevention. It is also a good source of medium chain triglycerides (MCT) and monounsaturated fatty acids (MUFA) that help with belly fat loss. Here is a list of dairy products for your daily consumption:

Milk (full fat D)	Ricotta	Butter Milk
Half and Half	Cottage cheese	Kefir
Heavy Cream	Khoa (Indian)	Sour Cream
Cheese	Paneer (Indian)	Cream Cheese

Lentils, Pulses, Legumes, and Select Grains

Lentils, pulses, and legumes are a rich source of plant protein. Most of these don't have all the essential amino acids, so it's a good idea to mix a few of them together since they will complement one other's protein profile to form a complete protein. They are also a good source of fiber and essential antioxidants. Whole grains (except modern wheat, rice, and corn) are also rich in fiber and certain proteins. Quinoa is technically not a grain but is marketed as such and has a complete amino acid profile, so it makes a healthy fat-burning food. Some of these can be sprouted, which boosts their nutritional value even further. Here is the list for your pantry.

- Green gram (Mung bean)
- Chickpeas
- Bengal Gram
- Kidney beans
- Fava beans
- Black Gram (Udad)
- Field bean (Val)
- Pigeon peas
- Moth bean
- Pink lentil (Masoor)
- Azuki Beans
- Navy Beans
- Barley
- Buckwheat (Kuttu)
- Quinoa
- Freekeh
- Einkorn

Meats, Poultry, Eggs, and Seafood for Looking Flat-Belly Good

Foods in this category are all without carbohydrates, so are prime foods for weight loss. They are also rich in thermogenic protein and healthy fats and many other essential vitamins and minerals. Make sure they are free pasture and minimally processed, which means sausages, bologna, pepperoni, and many processed deli meats are to be avoided. Make sure the fish is cold deep-sea variety and not the farmed variety. Farmed fish is fed the genetically modified grain chow that skews their omega-6/omega-3 fatty acid ratio.

The other drawback of farmed fish, poultry, and cattle is that they are kept in a restricted confined environment so they have high levels of stress hormones, which directly enter our body when we eat these sources of food.

Appendix B

Vegetarian Sources of Protein

Good protein doesn't always have to come from animal sources. This section contains information about plant proteins that can rival the best animal proteins.

Lacto-ovo vegetarians are often faced with a choice of eating eggs and/or dairy for complete sources of protein. Most of the vegetarian sources of proteins are lacking in certain amino acids that make them "incomplete." This makes the protein less bioavailable for the body to use. Vegetarians and vegans need not despair as there are good sources of protein from plant-based foods and here I list some of them.

Protein consists of 21 amino acids that are considered building blocks to form complete protein. Out of the 21, nine are considered essential since the human body cannot make them and so have to be ingested from dietary sources. All animal sources of protein are considered "complete" since they have the full spectrum of amino acids, while most plant sources are considered "incomplete" since they are missing one or more of the essential amino acids. Usually complementary vegetarian sources can be combined to get the complete amino acid spectrum. Rice and black beans are good examples. Rice has all the amino acids except methionine and black beans are a rich source of methionine. Combined, they form complete protein. Methionine is also found in nuts and seeds and some greens (spinach, watercress) so combining them with rice will make complete protein.

There are several vegetarian sources of complete protein like quinoa, soy, chia, pistachios, and others. However, I don't recommend eating soy-based protein mainly due to the high content of phytoestrogens, which are essentially estrogen-mimicking compounds. We already have too much of those in our processed diet and we certainly should avoid as much as we can. Men especially shouldn't touch soy-based anything with a 10-foot pole unless they want to grow man-boobs (gynecomastia). Plus, 95% of soy-based foods are made from GMO soybeans, which is another big unknown in terms of the harm it can do. Finally, why resort to soy when there are much better and healthier sources of good protein?

Table 1, below, shows plant sources of complete protein. The Amino Acid Profile (AAP) score is a qualitative measure of the completeness of a particular source of protein. A score of 100 or more implies that the food is a complete source of protein, while a score of less than 100 means its incomplete (deficient in one or more amino acids). I put in egg for comparison and because it's regarded as the gold standard of protein. You can see that some of the vegetarian sources are almost as good as eggs and certainly better than dairy. So if you are a vegetarian and are concerned about protein intake (and you should be), include some of these high-quality sources of protein in your diet. Stick to the ones with an AAP score of 100-plus. Some of the vegetarian sources like seeds and avocados not only provide high-quality protein but also a healthy dose of omega-3 fatty acids.

Food	AAP score	Food	AAP score
Egg	145	Rice + Kidney Beans	90
Pumpkin/Squash seeds	136	Cheese	85
Avocados	129	Whole milk	85
Spinach	120	Yogurt	84
Chia Seeds	115	Mung beans	83
Broccoli	112	Long grain brown rice	75
Hemp Seeds	>110	Long grain white rice	71
Pistachios	110	Wheat gluten	55
Soy*	108	Almonds	55
Chestnuts	107	Walnuts	55
Quinoa	106	Pasta	37
Rice + Black beans	103	Bread	35
Split pea	102		

Table 1: Plant-based sources of protein along with their AAP score.

Not only does protein help boost our metabolism, but it is also essential to maintaining muscle mass, which is crucial to maintaining a high basal metabolic rate (BMR).

The metabolic advantage that comes with substituting some of the carbohydrate calories with high-quality protein is crucial to losing those extra pounds and keeping them off. Additionally, if you can get those protein calories from high-quality plant sources (like hemp, chia, walnuts, etc.) you get the added benefit of balancing out your omega-6/omega-3 profile for better overall health.

Appendix C

Glycemic Index of Common Foods

This section has a list of glycemic index of common foods arranged in increasing GI value. A GI value of 55 or lower is considered low, while a GI of 55-70 is considered moderate and anything higher than 70 is considered high GI. The lower the GI the better it is for health.

Arranged in increasing GI value.

Food	GI Value	Food	GI Value
Nepal prickly pear cactus	7	Grapefruit	25
Mulga seed (Acacia aneura)	8	Lentils, red	25
Black bean seed	8	Mesquite cakes	25
Bengal gram dal (Chana dal)	8	Mung bean noodles	26
Yogurt, low fat, artificially sweet	14	Spaghetti, protein enriched	27
Soya beans, canned	14	Milk + 30 g bran	27
Peanuts	15	Milk, full fat	27
Acorns stewed with venison	16	Chick pea flour (besan chapatti) bread	27
Soya beans	18	Beans, dried, not specified	28
Rice bran	19	Sausages	28
Red kidney beans (Rajma)	19	Lentils, not specified	29
Cherries	22	Kidney beans	29
Fructose	22	Lentils, green	29
Peas, dried	22	Black beans	30
Milk, chocolate, artificially sweet	24	Soy milk	30
Brown beans (South African)	24	Butter beans + 5 g. sucrose	30
Barley, pearled	25	Oat bran & honey Loaf	30

Food	GI Value
Butter beans + 10 g. sucrose	31
Apricots, dried	31
Butter beans	31
Split peas, yellow, boiled	32
Milk, skim	32
Lima beans, baby, frozen	32
Fettuccine	32
Mars® M&Ms (peanut)	32
Nutella® spread(Ferrero)	32
Yogurt, low fat, fruit sugar sweet	33
Chick peas (garbanzo beans)	33
Mixed Grain Bread	34
Milk, chocolate, sugar sweetened	34
Kidney beans, autoclaved	34
Cheeky yam	34
Vermicelli	35
Yogurt, unspecified	36
Lima beans broth	36
Dates	36
Spaghetti, boiled 5 min	36
Pear, fresh	38
Spaghetti, whole meal	37
Apple	38
Navy beans	38
Tomato Soup	38
Corn tortilla	38
Brown beans (Mexican)	38
Green gram (mung beans)	38
Fish fingers	38
Barley kernel bread	39
Plum	39
Pinto beans	39
Kellogg's® All-Bran Fruit 'n Oats	39
Carrots, cooked	39
Ravioli, durum, meat filled	39
Mars® Snickers Bar	40
Apple juice	41

Food	GI Value
Chick peas, curry, canned	41
Wheat kernels	41
Black-eyed beans	41
Spaghetti, white	41
Peach, fresh	42
Chick peas, canned	42
Milk + custard + starch + sugar	43
Barley chapatti	43
Black gram	43
Bush honey, sugar bag	43
Fruit Loaf Bread	43
Orange	44
Pear, canned	44
Lentil soup, canned	44
Sweet potato	44
Pinto beans, canned	45
Carrot juice	45
Macaroni	45
Yakult (fermented milk)	45
Romano beans	46
Linguine	46
Rice, instant, boiled 1 minute	46
Cake, sponge	46
Rye kernel bread	46
Grapes	46
Pineapple juice	46
Black gram dal with semolina	46
Bread (Acacia coriacea)	46
Cake, banana, made with sugar	47
Fruit loaf (bread)	47
Ploughman's Loaf (bread)	47
Peach, canned	47
Instant noodles	47
Bunya nut pine	47
Oat bran bread	48
Bulgur	48
Rice, parboiled	48

Food	GI Value
Peas, green	48
Mixed grain bread	48
Rice, parboiled, high amylose	48
Grapefruit juice	48
Baked beans, canned	48
VO2 Max Energy Bar (chocolate; Mars®)	48
Porridge (oatmeal)	49
Red River Cereal®	49
Chocolate	49
Jams and marmalades	49
Pumpernickel	50
Ice cream, low fat	50
Tortellini, cheese	50
Barley, cracked	50
Dates (barhi)	50
Yam	51
Horse gram	51
Orange juice	52
Kidney beans, canned	52
Lentils, green, canned	52
Boost (Vanilla) meal	53
Bulgur bread	53
Bran Buds	53
Kiwifruit	53
Cake, pound	54
Wheat, quick cooking	54
Banana	54
Potato crisps	54
Bengal gram dal with semolina	54
Taro	54
Butter beans + 15 g. sucrose	54
Linseed rye bread	55
Oat bran	55
Buckwheat	55
Sweet corn	55
Rice, specialty	55

Food	GI Value
Spaghetti, durum	55
Kellogg's® Honey Smacks	55
Cake, banana, made without sugar	55
Rice, brown	55
Oatmeal cookies	55
Rich Tea® cookies	55
Fruit cocktail	55
Popcorn	55
Muesli	56
Mango	56
Sultanas	56
Potato, white, not specified, boiled	56
Rice, wild, Saskatchewan	57
Potato, new	57
Whole green gram	57
Kellogg's® Mini-Wheats (whole wheat)	57
Power bar (Power foods)	58
Met-Rx® (Vanilla) meal	58
Pita bread, white	57
Apricots, fresh	57
Bajra (millet)	57
Honey	58
Bran Chex®	58
Rice, white	58
Rice, white, high amylose	58
Rice vermicelli	58
Boost® High Protein (Vanilla) meal	59
Pastry	59
Digestives	59
Kellogg's® Just Right	59
Potato, white, Ontario	60
Pizza, cheese	60
Split pea soup	60
Ice cream	61
Muesli Bars	61
Potato, canned	61

Food	GI Value
Mars® Kudos Whole Grain Bars (choc chip)	61
Cytomax® (Orange)	62
Muffins	62
Shredded wheat meal	62
Maize chapatti	62
Green gram dal with semolina	62
Potato, Prince Edward Island®, boiled	63
Apricots, canned, syrup	64
Shortbread	64
Raisins	64
Beets	64
Mars® Bar	64
Power aid (Orange)	65
Rye flour bread	64
Semolina bread	64
Macaroni and Cheese	64
Black bean soup	64
Sucrose	64
Cake, flan	65
Oat kernel bread	65
Couscous	65
High fiber rye crispbread	65
Rock melon (muskmelon, cantaloupe)	65
Potato, steamed	65
Barley, rolled	66
Cordial, orange	66
Rice, Mahatma® Premium	66
Pineapple	66
Green pea soup, canned	66
Semolina	66
Cake, angel food	67
Barley flour bread	67
Arrowroot	67
Gnocchi	67
XLR8® (Orange)	68
Croissant	67
Grape-nuts	67
Breton® Wheat Crackers	67
Stoned Wheat Thins®	67
Soft drink, Fanta®	68
M'fino wild greens	68
Varagu millet	68
Breadfruit	68
Wheat bread, high fiber	68
Crumpet	69
Cornmeal	69
Mars® Skittles	69
Wheat bread, whole meal flour	69
Shredded Wheat	69
Kellogg's® Mini-Wheats (blackcurrant)	69
Power bar (Chocolate)	69
Melba toast	70
Cream of Wheat	70
Wheat Biscuits	70
Sao	70
Beans, dried, P. vulgaris	70
Potato mashed	70
Life Savers®	70
Fruit leather	70
Banana, unripe, steamed 1 hr.	70
Tapioca, steamed 1 hr.	70
Millet	71
Maize meal porridge, unrefined	71
Wheat bread, white	71
Golden grahams	71
Water crackers	71
Sultana Bran	71
Bagel, white	72
Watermelon	72
Swede (rutabaga)	72
Kaiser rolls	73
Potato, boiled, mashed	73
Met-Rx® bar (Vanilla)	74

Food	GI Value
Whole-wheat snack bread	74
Puffed wheat	74
Corn chips	74
Ensure® (Vanilla) meal	75
Bread stuffing	74
Cheerios®	74
Graham wafers	74
Maize meal porridge, refined	74
Castanospermum austral	74
Corn Bran	75
French fries	75
Pumpkin	75
Donut	76
Waffles	76
Breakfast bar	76
Rice, Pedle	76
Optifuel™ meal	78
Coco pops	77
Vanilla wafers	77
Rice cakes	77
Jowar	77
Green gram dal + paspalum scorbic	78
White Bread	78
Broad beans (fava beans, fool, foul)	79
PR Bar® (Cookies 'N Cream)	81
Post® Flakes	80
Rice, Sunbrown™ Quick	80
Jelly beans	80
Tapioca, boiled with milk	81
Puffed crispbread	81
Pretzels	81
Rice Krispies	82
Team	82
Potato, microwaved	82
Corn Chex	83
Potato, instant	83
Cornflakes	83

Food	GI Value
Potato, baked	85
Ragi (or Raggi)	86
Crispix™	87
Rice, Calrose	87
Rice, parboiled, low amylose	87
Gatorade® (Orange)	89
GatorPro® (Chocolate) meal	89
Rice, white, low amylose	88
Rice Chex	89
Rice Bubbles	90
Rice, instant, boiled 6 min	90
Wheat bread, gluten free	90
Cactus jam	91
Rice pasta, brown	92
Lucozade®	95
French baguette	95
Glucose	96
Parsnips	97
GatorLode® (Orange)	100
Clif bar® (Cookies & Cream)	101
Glucose tablets	102
Maltose	105
Tofu frozen dessert, non-dairy	115

Appendix D
The Skinny on Fat

"No diet will remove all the fat from your body because the brain is entirely fat. Without a brain, you might look good, but all you could do is run for public office."

George Bernard Shaw

In this section, you will see:

- Fat is essential to good health.
- The ratio of omega-6/omega-3 fats in your diet matters more than the absolute quantity of fat.

The last few decades have seen the demonization of fat, the invention of the USDA food pyramid, and a mistaken understanding of the role fat and carbohydrates play in our bodies. These unfortunate developments continue to be presented as fact, and as a result, we become fatter and sicker year by year.

In this section, you will learn accurate, up-to-date information on the surprising importance of fat in a healthy diet.

Here is the bottom line: fat is not only *essential* for healthy, long-term weight loss, but it also helps protect us from numerous pathogens and a host of chronic degenerative diseases such as cancers and mental disorders.

Fat is the basic building block of all cell membranes. Fat from diet is broken down into fatty acids and these fatty acids are incorporated into a double layer (lipid-bilayer), along with cholesterol, around the cell. This forms the cell membrane. This membrane acts as a physical barrier that separates the inner contents of the cell from its external environment. The cell membrane has several (protein) receptors attached to it to facilitate the transport of vital nutrients (oxygen, glucose etc.) in and out of cells. Not only this, but fat also facilitates the communication between other cells; for example, neurotransmitter receptors found in nerve cell membranes are used to communicate with other nerve cells. Apart from this, fat is also used to transport fat-soluble vitamins (A, D, E, and K) throughout our body.

Saturated vs. Unsaturated Fat

However, not all fats are the same. There are two broad classes of fats; saturated and unsaturated. Saturated fats are solids at room temperature and unsaturated fats are liquid. This is due to the difference in atomic structure. Saturated fats, also known as Saturated Fatty Acids (SFA), are dense, completely saturated with hydrogen atoms. Unsaturated fats are further subdivided into polyunsaturated fatty acids and monounsaturated fatty acids. Polyunsaturated Fatty Acids (PUFA) or oils have a less dense structure with (more than one) double bonds between the carbon atoms while Monounsaturated Fatty Acids (MUFA) have one double bond in the carbon chain. The double bonds in the carbon chain cause a "kink" in the otherwise straight carbon-carbon chain which makes it less densely packed. Each of these different types of fats is used for different purposes by the body.

Saturated fat packs densely and provides rigidity to cell membranes and helps protect cells from invading pathogens, while unsaturated fats provide fluidity to the cell membranes. Membrane fluidity is important for cell response to various external stimuli and cell signaling (communication between cells). Cell signaling governs tissue repair, immunity, and overall growth and development.

In this book, I use the term "fat" to mean both saturated and unsaturated fats. The chemical structure of these fats is shown in Figure 16

The cells of our body need both types of fat to function properly. For example, brain and nerve cells don't regenerate the same way as the cells found around other parts of our body (like skin and muscle cells) do, so they need to be more "robust" compared to the other cells. So these cells need to incorporate more saturated fat and cholesterol in their membranes. If you don't eat enough saturated fat and cholesterol, your brain cells will starve without these vital nutrients. It's been shown (and is no surprise) that cholesterol-lowering drugs cause memory loss and other problems of brain, like depression and violent behavior[71].

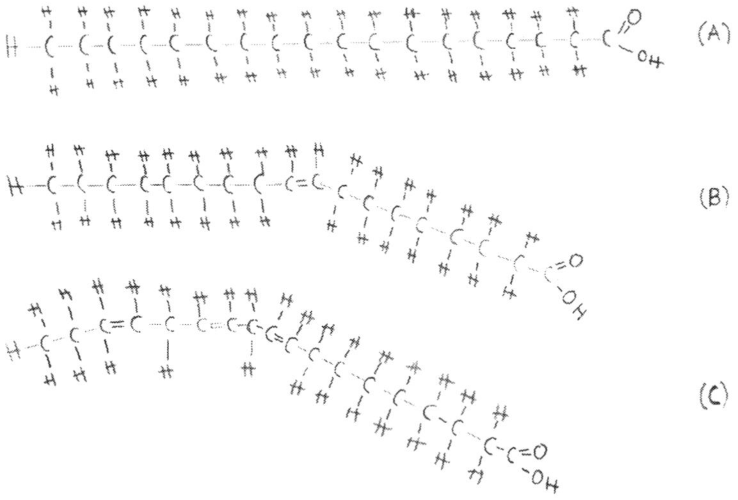

Figure 16: Saturated (A), Mono (B) and Polyunsaturated (C) fats.

Good health depends on having the right balance of both types of fats in your diet. This ensures a balance between rigidity and fluidity. Too much rigidity means the cells are unable to respond quickly to external stimuli, and cell communication becomes problematic. Too much fluidity means the cells are easily susceptible to invading pathogens.

Without this balance, the cell membrane is compromised and our cells can become handicapped, leading to lowered immunity, increased inflammation, inadequate cell signaling, and DNA dysfunction.

Three Sources of Fats

Most saturated fat comes from animal sources like meat, butter, lard, and dairy, while most unsaturated fat comes from plant sources like vegetable, fruit, nut, and seed oils.

A third kind of fat that was invented in response to the war against animal fats is called Trans-fat. This kind of fat is made by subjecting unsaturated vegetable oils to high temperatures in the presence of hydrogen and metal catalysts. This change in structure "saturates" the unsaturated fat, giving it all the properties of saturated fat without the burden of being animal fat. These types of artificial Trans-fats found in vegetable shortening and margarine found their way into all processed foods because they imparted a unique texture to food that was earlier imparted by cooking them with butter or lard (like grandma's delicious biscuits). Numerous studies have since shown that Trans-fats actively contribute to many lifestyle diseases, including heart disease, cancer, depression, and obesity, specifically belly fat. Despite its negative effects, Trans-fats are still found in almost all bakery items (cakes, pastries, cookies, etc.) and the majority of the processed foods on your market shelves and fast-food restaurants. According to the Independent Institute of Medicine, there is no safe level of consumption of Trans-fat[72], meaning the only safe level is zero[D]!

Omegas: The Balancing Act for Good Health

Further distinctions between unsaturated fatty acids are the omega-6 (also labeled as n-6) and omega-3 (also labelled at n-3) fatty acids. These fats are termed essential fatty acids (EFA) after scientists found that rats on a fat-free diet couldn't survive. These fatty acids play a vital role in cell and hormone function via the action of super hormones called *eicosanoids*. *Eicosanoids* (from Greek 'eikosa,' meaning 20) are formed from 20 carbon chain molecules present in certain fats. They are very short-lived signaling molecules that are capable of forming in every single cell of your body for "signaling" or "cueing" the action of hormones on them. In that sense, these are super-hormones that control the action of hormones. They first appeared in living cells 550 million years ago. There are no special glands that secrete these super-hormones as they can be secreted at the site of use by every single cell. *Eicosanoids* are created and used up in a matter of seconds and are not transported long distances in the body, yet, they play a vital role in inflammation, immunity, regulation of blood pressure, blood clotting, control of reproductive processes and tissue growth. In one word, they are pretty darn IMPORTANT!

D Many food labels will read "zero Trans-fats" even though they contain hydrogenated or partially hydrogenated fats. This is because FDA allows Trans-fats less than 0.5g/serving to be labeled as "zero Trans-fats." Eating multiple servings of these foods over the course of the day could still result in a substantial consumption of Trans-fats.

These tiny "switches" were first discovered in the 1930s in the prostate gland and hence were given the name Prostaglandin. These prostaglandins were isolated and purified and their structures and mechanisms were understood in the early 1960s. A decade later another eicosanoid, Thromboxane A2, a powerful platelet-aggregating agent, and prostacyclin, its antagonist, were discovered. In 1971, John Vane discovered how acetyl salicylic acid (the wonder drug aspirin) inhibited the synthesis of eicosanoids and was awarded the Nobel Prize in medicine in 1982 for discovering the role played by eicosanoids in human disease.

What is the link between eicosanoids and fat? Well, fat in our diet is converted to fatty acids and some of these fatty acids (EFAs) are also 20 carbons long. These form the eicosanoid building blocks. EFAs cannot be synthesized in the body and have to be ingested from dietary sources. Omega-3 (n-3) and omega-6 (n-6) fatty acids both belong to this class of fatty acids. The details of how eicosanoids are formed from EFAs is beyond the scope of this book, but readers interested in reading more about it can refer to the section on further references.

Staying pertinent to this discussion, I'll only state that there are four main kinds of eicosanoids: prostaglandins, prostacyclins, thromboxanes, leukotrienes. Although you will hear things like "good" and "bad" eicosanoids, I don't subscribe to those generalizations as I think everything our bodies make is for a reason and it is neither "good" nor "bad". Good health is a state of balance between all the subsystems in the body and eicosanoids are no exception. Its only when there is a shift in that balance that causes "good" and "bad" effects. For example, it is known that thromboxanes are eicosanoids that cause blood platelets to clump together. There is an optimum level of thromboxane in the body, but when the balance shifts one way or another, problems happen. For example if the balance shifts toward higher levels of thromboxane, there is more platelet aggregation and for a patient with heart disease, it could spell stroke. On the other hand, if the balance shifts toward the low side, then a person could bleed to death from a minor cut.

Omega-3 fatty acids are vital in the creation of docosahexaenoic acid (DHA) that forms the basic building block of the human brain and the cerebral cortex. Many studies now show that DHA is *the* most important fat that is required for proper brain development and cognitive functioning in growing kids[73, 74]. So it is quite clear that the omega-3 fatty acids play a vital role in the development of the human brain.

Omega-3 creates the eicosanoids that play a vital role in inflammation, immunity, regulation of blood pressure, blood clotting, control of reproductive processes, and tissue growth. Omega-6 fatty acids make the eicosanoids that play a crucial role in increasing inflammation and clotting and are responsible for the body's repair and healing mechanisms at the cellular level. A balance between the consumption of these two can't be overstated.

For example, omega-3 forms the hormones that inhibit blood clotting and are responsible for relaxing our arteries (also known as vasodilation), causing a drop in blood pressure. Omega-6, on the other hand, forms the hormones that increase blood clotting and are responsible for constricting our arteries (also known as vasoconstriction), and injury healing via inflammation. If the balance shifts more toward omega-3, our blood-clotting capability is compromised and we could bleed to death from a paper cut. If the balance shifts more toward omega-6, a plaque rupture inside an artery (that provides blood to the heart or brain) will cause a clot blockage in the artery, cutting off blood supply to that part of the heart or brain. This will cause a heart attack or stroke. Figure 17 shows a schematic representation of what effects are seen in the body with increasing consumption of one omega over the other.

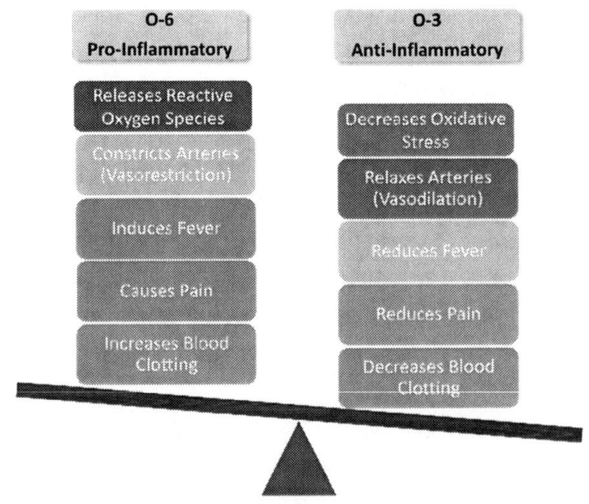

Figure 17: Schematic representation of balance between the two omegas. On the left are the effects of o-6 and on the right are effects of o-3. When the consumption of one type of omega goes up, so does its effect on the body[75].

The other problem is that both omega-6 and omega-3 fatty acids are competing for the same precursors that form these vital hormones. So an excess of one type of omega will suppress the formation of hormones that are made from the other type of omega, causing an imbalance in the production of these essential hormones.

> Humans have evolved on an omega-6/omega-3 ratio of 1:1 – 4:1

The balance of omega fats in our body is measured in terms of the ratio of omega-6/omega-3. The higher this ratio, the more your balance shifts toward inflammatory conditions shown in Figure 17. Humans have evolved on an omega-6/omega-3 ratio of 1:1 – 4:1, and experts agree that this is the ideal ratio to prevent most lifestyle diseases and cancers. Given the virtual epidemic of obesity and lifestyle diseases in the United States, it's not surprising the typical Western diet has a ratio of approximately 16/1. According to the latest research[76, 77],

> *"...a high Omega-6/Omega-3 ratio, as is found in today's Western diets, promotes the pathogenesis of many diseases, including cardiovascular disease, cancer, and inflammatory and autoimmune diseases, whereas... increased levels of omega-3 PUFA [a low omega-6/omega-3 ratio] exerts suppressive effects."*

Furthermore, disease prevention studies have found that[78],

> *"In the secondary prevention of cardiovascular disease,* ***a ratio of 4/1 was associated with a 70% decrease in total mortality... The lower omega-6/omega-3 ratio in women with breast cancer was associated with decreased risk."*** (emphasis added)

Studies have also shown that omega-3 supplementation can be used to treat depression[79]. The brain is two-thirds fat and the synaptic membranes of brain cells and neurons contain high concentrations of DHA. Low blood concentrations of DHA result in low concentrations of cerebrospinal fluid, which has been linked to suicide and depression. Studies have also shown that a diet high in omega-6 (15% total energy intake) can increase levels of DNA damage which may then play a role in cancer cell growth[80].

We get too much omega-6 in our modern diets from vegetable oils such as soybean, grape-seed, corn, and sunflower oils. We need to reduce our consumption of vegetable oils and balance that with increased omega-3 fats from fatty cold-water fish, krill oil, free pasture eggs, grass-fed meat, and butterfat. Vegetarian sources of omega-3 are flax seeds, hemp oil, walnuts, and olive oil and canola oil (cold-pressed, unrefined).

The one important distinction between animal and vegetable sources of omega-3 is that animal sources contain DHA in its native form that is easily absorbed in the body (high bioavailability). Vegetable sources of omega-3 have to be converted to DHA in the human body and this conversion efficiency is typically less than 5%[81].

Table 2 lists the most common foods and oils with their ratios of omega-6/omega-3. Remember, a ratio of 4 or less is ideal.

Fish and meats	omega-6/omega-3 Ratio
Tuna, canned in water, drained	0.1
Cod, fresh and frozen, cooked	0.1
Mackerel, canned, drained	0.1
Bluefish, fresh and frozen, cooked	0.1
Smelt, Rainbow	0.1
Scallops, Maine, fresh and frozen, cooked	0.1
Salmon, cold water, fresh and frozen, cooked	0.2
Swordfish, fresh and frozen, cooked	0.2
Lobster, cooked	0.2
Salmon, canned, drained	0.4
Sardines, canned in oil, drained	2.2
Grass fed red meat (mixed cattle)	2.78
Grain Fed red meat (mixed cattle)	13.6

Nuts and Seeds	omega-6/omega-3 Ratio
Flax seeds	0.2
Linseed	0.24
Chia seeds	0.25
Hemp seeds	2.5
Walnuts	4.2
Pecans, dry roasted	22
Pistachios, roasted	55.3
Sesame seeds	55.7
Poppy seeds	96
Pumpkin seeds, shelled	107.8
Almonds, dry roasted#	-

Fats and Oils	omega-6/omega-3 Ratio
Cod liver oil	0.1
Sardine oil	0.1
Flax seed oil.	0.3
Ghee/butter (clarified butterfat)	1
Canola oil*	2.2
Hemp oil.	3
Walnut oil.	5.1
Soybean oil, un-hydrogenated.	7.5
Lard	10
Duck fat	12
Avocado oil	13
Extra Virgin Olive Oil	13
Olive oil	13.4
Chicken fat	17
Sunflower oil	39
Palm oil	46
Cottonseed oil	47.8
Corn oil	55.5
Safflower oil	133
Sesame oil	137
Grapeseed oil	676
Peanut oil#	-

Table 2: List of foods containing fat with their omega-6/omega-3 ratios.

Note:

*Oils are cold-pressed and unrefined.

#Contains no Omega-3 so technically the ratio is infinite.

Source: Tufts University School of Medicine.

We have come a long way in understanding the role of fat from the days when fat was regarded as the sole cause of obesity. Today, fat is regarded as a key nutrient for the human body. Scientists at the 2008 Food and Nutrition Conference in Geneva[82] concluded:

> *"We now have a better understanding of how fats and fatty acids are metabolized and utilized in the body, how they alter cell membrane function, how they control gene transcription and expression, and how they*

interact with each other. Fats and fatty acids should now be considered as key nutrients that affect early growth and development and nutrition-related chronic disease later in life. For example, specific n-3 and n-6 fatty acids are essential nutrients and also, as part of the overall fat supply, may affect the prevalence and severity of cardiovascular disease, diabetes, cancer and age-related functional decline. Dietary fats provide the medium for the absorption of fat-soluble vitamins; are a primary contributor to the palatability of food; and are crucial to proper development and survival during the early stages of life-embryonic development and early growth after birth on through infancy and childhood. Thus, the role of essential fatty acids during pregnancy and lactation is highlighted, and the role of long-chain n-3 fatty acids as structural components for the development of the brain and central nervous system is now accepted…."

Apart from important body functions, fat is also essential for healthy skin, hair, and vision. Without fat, our brain and central nervous system would stop working, our cells would perish and we would have no immunity from external pathogens. In a word, without fat, we die!

What About Vegetable Oil?

Omega-6 fatty acids, abundant in vegetable oils, are pro-inflammatory. Inflammation is commonly considered a bad thing today, yet some amount is necessary to the healthy functioning of our immune systems. Unfortunately, overreliance on vegetable oils results in too much omega-6, pushing our bodies into a chronic inflammation state. This leads to a host of problems, ranging from allergic reaction to arthritis to atherosclerosis and even some forms of cancer[83, 84]. Studies have also shown that overreliance on vegetable oils may increase the likelihood of breast cancer in post-menopausal women[85] and prostate cancer in men[86].

The other problem with vegetable oils is the modern methods of extracting it, which employ high temperatures and pressures in excess of 2000 Centigrade and several tons/inch and typically use industrial solvents (hexane, sodium hydroxide) to extract the last trace of oil. Furthermore, chemical bleach is used to lighten the natural color of oil to give the impression that the oil is 'light' in calories and healthier than comparable animal fats (all fats have 9 calories/gram, irrespective of their color or origin). The thermal and chemical processing in the presence of light and oxygen damages (oxidizes) the fragile carbon-carbon bonds of the polyunsaturated fatty acids, creating dangerous free radicals. So any beneficial properties of omega-3 in refined vegetable oils are rendered useless and toxic even before the oil hits the store shelves.

Vegetable oil extraction that uses expellers to press out the virgin oil from the seeds at room temperature and filter the oil for particulates retains most of the beneficial fats and antioxidants in vegetable oil. This type of virgin oil, stored in dark bottles in cooler temperatures, will retain all the healthy properties of omega-3 for a long time. Cold-pressed flax seed, extra virgin olive, walnut, and hemp oils are best used uncooked in salad dressings. Other oils such as cold-pressed avocado, sesame, etc., can be used for minimal cooking and light frying. For deep-frying, saturated fats like ghee (clarified butterfat), coconut, and palm oil are the best. Refined avocado oil is also suited to deep-frying as it has a high smoke point.

Appendix E

Cholesterol: The 20th Century Bugaboo

"Too often we enjoy the comfort of opinion without the discomfort of thought."

John F. Kennedy

In this section, you will see:

- How the misguided war on cholesterol has caused more harm than good.
- Why cholesterol is beneficial to health.

Whenever we hear the word "cholesterol," we automatically think of heart disease. Ever since Ancel Keys published his Minnesota Businessmen Study[87] in 1963 and his Seven Countries Study shortly thereafter, showing an apparent correlation between consumption of fat and the incidence of heart disease, we have been obsessed with eliminating cholesterol and saturated fats from our diets.

Ever since then, cholesterol went from being a natural substance synthesized in our body to becoming the biggest killer of humankind in the 20th century. I don't want to go into the history of how the cholesterol-heart disease hypothesis came into existence, but for more information please refer to the further reading section.

Let's take a closer look at this mysterious substance and see if the real facts about cholesterol hold up to the negative hyperbole.

What is Cholesterol Anyway?

Cholesterol belongs to a class of waxy substances called sterols from which all steroid hormones are made. It is used by the male testes to make testosterone and by the female ovaries to make estrogen. Cholesterol is also used to make vitamin D and bile acids that are used to digest food. Cholesterol, along with fat, also forms an integral part of cell membranes and helps regulate membrane fluidity. Without cholesterol, membranes would be too fluid and be easily destroyed with a change in external environment (like temperature). Cells that need to be more environmentally robust, like brain and central nervous system cells, use more cholesterol in their membranes than, say, cells in your muscle tissue.

Any cell of the body is capable of making the cholesterol it needs, but the liver is especially efficient at churning out large quantities of cholesterol that can be transported around the body for use by other tissues and organs. The body's production of cholesterol is tightly regulated, which means the body maintains a certain "baseline" level. If you get a lot of cholesterol in your diet, the liver makes less of it, and vice versa. Typical daily requirement of cholesterol is anywhere from 1000 mg to 1800mg.

Many Forms of Lipoproteins

Cholesterol is insoluble in blood. To reach its destination, cholesterol is packed into tiny little molecules known as lipoproteins; a combination of lipid (fat) and protein. These lipoproteins filled with cholesterol circulate freely in blood to reach the point of use.

Lipoproteins come in many sizes and flavors, but the two most important ones that we hear about are low-density lipoprotein (LDL or bad cholesterol) and high-density lipoprotein (HDL or good cholesterol). From a strict biochemical standpoint, these molecules aren't even cholesterol. LDL is what transports cholesterol to the point of use (including the arteries where it forms plaque) while HDL is what ferries excess cholesterol back to the liver for recycling.

> there is no "good" or "bad" cholesterol

You will often read about HDL being a "vacuum cleaner" of cholesterol, giving us the impression that it sucks up cholesterol from your clogged arteries and unclogs them. Nothing of this sort happens once plaque is formed in your arteries, because the role of LDL is simple: dump cholesterol into the arterial walls and let the cells take care of it. But once this cholesterol is captured inside of plaque, it isn't easily given up in order for HDL to carry it back to the liver. As a result, atherosclerotic plaque only gets worse with time, and rarely regresses.

Atherosclerosis is a race between HDL and LDL to shuttle cholesterol back and forth from target organs. A higher level of LDL promotes atherosclerosis while a higher level of HDL prevents it. This is why the ratio of LDL/HDL is a better predictor of heart disease risk than total cholesterol level. You could have a high total cholesterol level, but as long as it's being efficiently transported and recycled, it poses no threat to heart health. In other words, there is no "good" or "bad" cholesterol. Cholesterol has a purpose and LDL and HDL are merely vehicles for transporting it within our bodies.

The Saturated Fat Conundrum

Animal fats are a rich source of saturated fatty acids (SFA). Short-term feeding studies have shown that saturated fats increase total cholesterol levels, which is why they were thought of as being a contributor to heart disease.

More recently, though, it has been found that ,even though saturated fats increase total cholesterol levels, they increase both LDL and HDL levels, so the ratio of LDL/HDL is more or less preserved[88, 89]. Furthermore, saturated fat has been shown to increase the quantity of large buoyant LDL (lbLDL), which is NOT associated with plaque formation[90]. The other LDL type, which is small dense LDL (sdLDL), is shown to be plaque forming[91] because it easily penetrates the artery walls (where it contributes to plaque formation). The small size of sdLDL particles also makes it highly susceptible to oxidization, which makes it sticky. It has been shown that this oxidation of LDL plays an important role in the initiation and progression of plaque formation[92]. Individuals with higher levels of sdLDL have more than a three-fold risk for heart disease[93].

even though saturated fats increase total cholesterol levels, they increase both LDL and HDL levels

Now here is the bigger puzzle: some recent studies have noted an *inverse correlation* between saturated fat intake and overall all-cause mortality (not just from heart disease). One such large study[94] noted:

> *"...decreasing SFA intake by increasing PUFA was significantly positively associated with stroke mortality..."*

In other words, substituting saturated fats with vegetable oils (PUFA) caused an increase in stroke mortality!

Another study[95] noted a decrease in the risk for Ischemic Stroke with increasing saturated fat consumption. Another study[96] with a 14-year follow up period concluded that:

> *"Intakes of red meats, high fat dairy products, nuts, and eggs were also not appreciably related to risk of stroke. These findings do not support associations between intake of total fat, cholesterol, or specific types of fat and risk of stroke in men."*

In an article from 2013 titled "*Saturated fat is not the major issue*," published in the British Medical Journal[97], Dr. Aseem Malhotra, a London-based cardiologist, noted:

> *"The mantra that saturated fat must be removed to reduce the risk of cardiovascular disease has dominated dietary advice and guidelines for almost four decades. Yet scientific evidence shows that this advice has, paradoxically,* ***increased*** *our cardiovascular risks"* (Emphasis added)

Could Our "Heart Healthy" Low-Fat Diet be Causing Heart Disease?

So far, we have seen how our recommended low-fat/high-carbohydrate diet is responsible in making us overweight, and indirectly contributing to metabolic syndrome, diabetes, and heart disease. But could this diet also be modifying our blood composition in such a way to be directly responsible for heart disease?

Randomized double blind studies of low-fat/high-carbohydrate and high-fat/low-carbohydrate diets have shown that a low-fat (high carbohydrate) diet increases the production of dangerous sdLDL while the high-fat (low-carbohydrate) diet increases the formation of benign lbLDL particles[98]. Metabolic syndrome arising from carbohydrate overconsumption also promotes the formation of sdLDL.

In another controlled study, subjects consuming a high-fat diet (61% calories from fat) showed lower triglycerides, lower blood sugar, increased HDL concentration, and increased LDL particle size (benign lbLDL type)[99]. On the other hand, subjects on a low-fat diet (32% fat calories) showed higher triglycerides, higher blood sugar, and even though their LDL levels were moderately lowered, the LDL particles reduced in size to the more dangerous sdLDL type.

Blood triglyceride levels are an independent (of cholesterol) predictor of the risk for heart disease. Increase in triglyceride levels is a well-documented effect of high-carbohydrate diets[100]. It seems like the low-fat/high-carbohydrate diets that were supposed to reduce our risk for heart disease might be responsible for giving us that heart attack.

Cholesterol-Heart Disease Hypothesis: A World of Paradoxes

Consider the following paradoxes that can't be explained by the cholesterol-heart disease hypothesis:

1) **Coconut oil paradox:** In a study[101], supplementation with 30ml coconut oil vs. soybean oil showed that coconut oil (which contains 86% saturated fat) improved the cholesterol profile (increased HDL, lowered LDL/HDL ratio) and decreased waist circumference (all three being markers for heart disease), while soybean oil decreased HDL, increased LDL, and didn't do anything for reducing waist circumference.

2) **Mother's milk paradox:** Mother's milk has 60% of calories as fat and cholesterol out of which about 37% is saturated fat. Formula is less than 30% fat and zero cholesterol. Observational studies have shown that infants fed mother's milk show lower levels of cholesterol, have a lower risk of type II diabetes, are leaner, and have lower BP as adults when

compared to infants who are fed formula[102]. Even carefully controlled randomized trials have shown that breast-fed infants had significantly lower blood pressure (BP), more favorable plasma lipid profile, and reduced leptin resistance at age of 13-15 years compared with those who were fed formula[103].

3) **Atkins Paradox:** A 2007 study at Stanford[104] compared four popular diets and their effect on obesity (body mass index, waist-to-hip ratio) and lipid profile (HDL, LDL, Triglycerides, BP, glucose). The diets compared were the Atkins diet, which was mostly a diet of fat and protein from animal sources, hence rich in saturated fat and cholesterol, the Zone diet, which is also low in carbohydrate but not as carbohydrate restrictive at the Atkins, the USDA diet, and the Ornish diet, the lowest fat and highest carbohydrate diet. And the winner turned out to be the Atkins diet! The Atkins diet not only caused the most weight loss but also improved the lipid profile the most. The Atkins diet group lost the most weight and showed the greatest reduction in body mass index and waist-to-hip ratio. Over a 12-month period, it also showed the greatest increase in HDL cholesterol, greatest reduction in BP, greatest reduction in fasting glucose, and greatest reduction in triglycerides. The lead on this trial, Dr. Christopher Gardner, who happens to be a vegetarian for 25 years, concluded that the healthiest diet turned out to be the Atkins diet full of red meat and saturated fat, and he called it "a bitter pill to swallow."

4) **The French Paradox:** The French eat a lot more saturated fat and cholesterol (from cheeses, organ meats, dairy, and red meat) compared to the average person in the UK and the USA, and have a higher average cholesterol (some in the 300 range), and yet the incidence of coronary heart disease is much lower in France compared to that in the UK and the USA[105]. The Swiss exhibit a similar trend.

5) **North vs. South India mortality from CHD:** South Indians are about 7 times more likely to die of heart attacks

compared to north Indians[106] even though the people in north eat 17 times more saturated fat, from clarified butterfat, cholesterol, and meats. The rate of diabetes is also higher in south Indians, who, by the way, are predominantly vegetarians.

6) **Low-cholesterol paradox:** This is a classic! Half the people who die of heart attacks have average to low cholesterol, so obviously cholesterol is not the reason for their heart attacks.

In Appendix G, you will see how oxidation and chronic inflammation are the real cause of heart disease. Cholesterol has been wrongly accused of causing heart disease. While cholesterol is found in plaque, it's an innocent bystander on the crime scene of heart disease.

Cholesterol has an important role to play in human health and the following sections explore the various benefits of cholesterol and why it's not a substance to be feared, but rather, revered.

The Risks of Low Cholesterol

Mother Nature didn't make cholesterol to be a toxic substance; otherwise, it would have been eliminated from our bodies a long time ago via positive natural selection. Cholesterol has a purpose to fulfill in our body and rather than trying to lower it via medications, it's best to understand the real cause of heart disease (described in Appendix G) and address that instead. In fact, having lower levels of cholesterol carry several risks, especially as we get older. Here are some of the risks associated with low cholesterol:

Cholesterol and the Brain

The role of cholesterol has profound implications for brain and nerve cell functionality and longevity. As noted earlier in this chapter, nerve and brain cells are the ones that use the most cholesterol since they don't regenerate like other cells and need to maintain their robustness. So what happens when cholesterol levels go down with, say, the use of cholesterol lowering (statin) drug? The result is the onset of nerve and brain cell death, due to which poor brain function, depression, memory loss, and suicidal tendencies increase and get worse as the dosage of statin is increased. In his book,

Lipitor, Thief of Memory: Statin Drugs and the Misguided War on Cholesterol, Dr. Duane Graveline talks about how the use of statins caused him to lose both short-term and long-term memory and how he eventually was diagnosed with transient global amnesia (TGA). Even the FDA acknowledged that statin use could result in loss of memory and predispose one to developing type II diabetes, along with the risk of liver and muscle damage[107].

The profound role of cholesterol in brain health can be understood by looking at the therapeutic value of ketogenic diets. A ketogenic diet (KD) is very high in saturated fats and cholesterol, mostly from butter, cheese, bacon and other red meats, with minimal carbohydrates and enough protein to sustain growth. Studies done at Johns Hopkins on the benefits of KD on the human brain[108]show that it can help with symptoms of epilepsy. In this study, the authors have shown how KD can help children with epilepsy. When other conventional medications for the treatment of epilepsy fail, a child is put on KD for a period of two years, and in most cases the child is fully cured. The study further went on to show that KD can provide symptomatic and disease-modifying activity in a broad range of neurodegenerative disorders, including Alzheimer's disease and Parkinson's disease, and may also be protective in traumatic brain injury and stroke. KD has also been shown to act as an antidepressant[109]. The Lucile Packard Children's Hospital Stanford has a wealth of information about KD and treatment for epilepsy in children[110].

There are other studies[111] that show that a deficiency of cholesterol hinders action with serotonin receptors in the brain, leading to autism spectrum disorders (ASD). They have shown that individuals treated with dietary supplementation of cholesterol display fewer autistic behaviors, infections, and symptoms of irritability and hyperactivity, with improvements in physical growth, sleep and social interactions. Other behaviors shown to improve with cholesterol supplementation include aggressive behaviors, self-injury and temper outbursts[112].

Cholesterol and Muscle

The effect of a low-cholesterol diet on muscle cells has been studied by researchers at the Texas A&M University [113].Various mechanisms of statin toxicity have been identified in the case of muscle cells. These factors reduce muscle mass, energy, vitality, and lead to general lack of fitness. In this study, they compared two groups of people on a strict exercise regimen, but one group was given statin drugs while the other was given a placebo. They found that the group that took cholesterol-lowering statin drugs had a lower muscle strength gain. Muscle fatigue and pain is a well-documented side effect of statin drugs. This could be related to lower production of testosterone, the main muscle-building hormone in the body.

Cholesterol and Cancer

Recent studies have found that having low cholesterol levels could be an indication of brewing cancer. Although there is no causal relationship established between a low cholesterol levels and the occurrence of cancer, several studies have shown that a low serum cholesterol level predates the development of cancer by several years. This correlation has been found to be true whether your cholesterol level is low due to medications or naturally so.

In two large studies[114, 115], 10,000 people (in each study) were divided into two groups. One group was put on cholesterol-lowering medication and the other group received the placebo pill. Both studies had a follow-up period of about five years. Average reduction of total cholesterol in the treatment groups was 9% and 11.6%. In both studies, more number of people in the treatment group who got the cholesterol lowering medication died of cancer and from coronary, cardiac, and non-cardiovascular deaths!

In another epidemiological study done in 1992[116] that sought answers to two basic questions:

a) Is having low serum cholesterol associated with increased risk of cancer?
b) Does reducing serum cholesterol increase the occurrence of cancer?

It was found that:

"Some elevated risk of cancer for males with low serum cholesterol levels has been noted: the median of the studies examined is consistent with a 30% increased risk..."

In aggregate, the trials of lipid-lowering interventions reviewed here show an increase in cancer occurrence (primarily mortality) of approximately 24% in the cholesterol-lowered groups... Recent evidence indicates that *products in the **cholesterol biosynthetic pathway** affect DNA replication and cell proliferation. These findings suggest a mechanism by which cholesterol lowering might accelerate the development of tumors already initiated.*" (emphasis added)

"Cholesterol biosynthetic pathway" modifiers refer to cholesterol-lowering medications.

Another recent meta-analysis published in 2011[117] had this to report:

"*...four controlled, randomized statin trials have resulted in a statistically significant increase of cancer in the treatment group; and several case–control and cohort studies have also shown a significant risk of cancer associated with statins... We identified nine cohort studies including more than 140,000 individuals, where **cancer was inversely associated with cholesterol** measured 10–30 years earlier.*" (emphasis added)

This meant, the lower your cholesterol levels, the higher your risk of developing cancer! The latest study[118] reported in 2012 states that:

"*There may be a link between low levels of "bad" low-density lipoprotein (LDL) cholesterol and increased cancer risk.*"

"Bad" cholesterol may not be that bad after all.

The famous Merck and Schering-Plough cholesterol-lowering drug Vytorin is being investigated for fraud across the country for increasing the risk of certain forms of cancer by 64%. The drug is very good at lowering LDL cholesterol but in doing so, it substantially increases the risk of some forms of cancer. There are numerous ongoing studies investigating the link between low LDL levels and the risk of developing cancer[119].

The relation between heart disease and high cholesterol has been so ingrained in our psyche that we never think of questioning this notion. Any mention of heart disease brings forth images of arteries clogged with cholesterol-rich plaque deposits; while that is partly true, it doesn't convey the full picture. The real mechanism of plaque formation is way more complex to be explained by the simple analogy of excess cholesterol depositing in our arteries. Appendix G discusses the real mechanism of plaque formation and heart disease.

The fact that cholesterol in our diet does not cause heart disease is being realized by nutrition experts. In fact, the 2015 dietary guidelines released by the USDA removed the longstanding recommendation on restricting the intake of dietary cholesterol by noting that:

"Cholesterol is not considered a nutrient of concern for overconsumption."

This should put to rest any fear that might come out of eating cholesterol and getting heart disease.

Appendix F

Beyond Weight Gain: How Sugar Causes Premature Aging

"Sugar is the new tobacco."

Cynthia Kenyon

In this section, you will see:

- How excess blood sugar contributes to many chronic diseases and premature aging.

The guy in the next cube at your office has a pronounced potbelly and even though he claims he is only 40, he looks more like a 60-year-old with receding hairline, dry scalp, and crow's feet around his eyes. His skin seems wrinkled and spotty, and every time you watch him climb stairs, he is huffing like a 60-year-old as he pauses to catch his breath. Sounds familiar? We all have come across a few such people that seem overly ripe for their age.

Are they lying about their age, or are they aging faster than they should? The answer lies in AGE, which is short for Advanced Glycation End-products.

Many of today's lifestyle diseases are a result of AGE, and in fact, normal ageing is also thought to happen due to the formation of AGE[120]. Diabetes is one such example of the direct result of AGE formation in our body.

AGE are formed when excess glucose attaches to either protein or fat. This process is called glycation. These glycated proteins and fats never get eliminated from our system and build up over time in the various organs and tissues.

The study of diabetes offers us a unique window into the ageing mechanism, as diabetics experience the most accelerated aging. Diabetics have impaired healing capability, they have organ failures more often, their vision fades faster, and their bones and skin deteriorate faster. In other words, they simply age faster.

Why AGE Makes You Age

We saw in Chapter 2 how insulin resistance and metabolic syndrome result in high levels of circulating blood glucose right after a meal and sometimes for prolonged periods thereafter. It is during this time that AGE formation happens. Free-floating glucose molecules in our blood attach spontaneously (without the need for any enzyme) to protein and fat molecules in the blood to form stable irreversible compounds. As these AGE compounds continue to build in our system and travel to various tissues and organs around the body, they cause rampant inflammation and impaired cellular function—and the result is premature and accelerated ageing.

There is some AGE formation due to the normal aging process and cannot be avoided, but in the presence of metabolic syndrome and poor eating habits, AGE formation is drastically exacerbated. Age researchers believe that the definitive biological marker to measure our biological age is to measure AGE[121]. So even though your office colleague's age is 40, he's been exposed to chronic levels of high sugar from poor eating and lifestyle choices. For all practical purposes, his tissues and organs have sustained AGE damage equivalent to what they would have sustained in 60 years. In other words, his biological age is 60, even though he is only 40 years old.

AGE and Disease

AGE accumulation has detrimental effects on the organs. Here are some of the detrimental effects:

1) Causes kidney failure (nephropathy)[122].

2) Causes oxidative damage to the pancreatic beta cells that produce insulin[123], causing diabetes.

3) Causes arterial stiffness leading to high blood pressure[124].

4) Causes oxidation in the endothelial lining of the arteries, which initiates inflammation leading to atherosclerosis[125].

5) Causes cerebral infarction and dementia in the brain[126].

6) Causes arterial fibrillation in the heart[127].

7) Causes retinopathy and macular degeneration in the retinal cells[128].

8) Causes the formation of wrinkles in skin by crosslinking to collagen and elastin.

In other words, AGE causes you to age faster (no pun intended)!

Birthday Cakes Cause AGE

While AGE can be produced in our body (endogenous), they can also come from external sources (exogenous). Food is the biggest source of exogenous AGE. Proteins and fats cooked at high temperatures in the presence of sugars can lead to AGE formation. Most barbequed and grilled meats coated with various barbeque sauces that have sugars or worse, High Fructose Corn Syrup (HFCS), are prone to AGE formation.

Most deep-fried carbohydrates are prone to AGE formation as well. Caramelization, which involves heating refined sugar to high temperatures to form caramel, is also loaded with AGE. Some fast-food makers add sugars to fried products to impart a golden brown color, which also produces AGE. Likewise, various bakery products (cakes, pastries, donuts) are a rich source of AGE[129]. So the more birthday cakes you have had in your life, the more AGE you have.

The Role of Fructose in Aging

One key culprit in causing accelerated glycation in our bodies is high-fructose corn syrup (HFCS), omnipresent in all sweetened beverages. Fructose, the type of sugar found in fruits, has a lower glycemic index so it is absorbed in the blood slower than simple glucose. This is because most fructose passes through the gut intact and it processed almost entirely in the liver. This is why fructose has been suggested as a sugar substitute for many diabetics. But studies have shown the rate of glycation of fructose is 10 times faster than glucose[130]. It is also suggested to be a liver toxin causing fatty liver disease in the long run. So you can see why HFCS used in almost all processed foods and beverages contribute to accelerated aging and many of today's lifestyle diseases. Fructose has also shown to cause leptin resistance in animal models[131].

High-sugar fruits like mangoes, pineapple, grapes, and others should also be eaten in moderation as well.

AGE Measurement to Measure Age

You might be wondering if it's possible to measure our blood levels of AGE to determine our biological age. The problem is that AGE measurement of blood sample doesn't necessarily reflect tissue age. Also, most direct measurements of AGE accumulation in the body are invasive, expensive, and time-consuming. One non-invasive method that is used for clinical evaluation is skin auto fluorescence (AF). Just like other tissue, skin also collects AGE radicals over time and these AGE radicals have a unique property that causes them to glow (fluoresce) in the dark. Skin AF involves radiating the skin with a special light that causes AGE to absorb the light and glow in the dark. The intensity of this glow is measured, and from this one can find out how much AGE accumulation has occurred.

Another method that doctors commonly prescribe to measure the amount of glycation in your blood is to measure your HbA1c (also known as A1c). This test measures how much of your hemoglobin is glycated. Since hemoglobin has a life of about three months (after which it's replaced by new hemoglobin), HbA1c gives you a cumulative measure of AGE for the past three months. A fasting blood sugar measurement, on the other hand, is of limited utility as it only gives your blood sugar level for a particular instant. The former reveals a lot more about your lifestyle and eating habits than the latter.

The next time your doctor orders blood work for you, make sure you ask for an HbA1c test. This is one of the most important numbers that indicate your potential risk for lifestyle diseases like diabetes and heart disease. A normal HbA1c level is below 5, meaning that less than 5% of your hemoglobin is glycated. This is the maximum amount of glycation that would happen in a healthy person. This corresponds to an average blood glucose level of 97 mg/dL. HbA1c between 5 and 6.5 is pre-diabetic and anything over 6.5 is diabetic, which corresponds to average blood sugar levels in excess of 140 mg/dL.

Eating a slice of bread will send your blood glucose level from a normal reading of less than 100 mg/dL to over 170 mg/dL in a matter of two hours. In most people with moderate insulin resistance, blood sugar levels of over 200 mg/dL 1-2 hours after a slice of bread are not unusual. So if a slice of bread can do that, you can imagine what that cake and soda pop does to your blood sugar levels. You do that often enough and rest assured, you will age at an accelerated rate.

Aging is the normal process of growing old, and our tissues deteriorate at a certain rate over time. This is unavoidable. But when we over-rely on easily digested carbohydrates to provide our nutritional needs, we induce an accelerated rate of deterioration on our tissues due to the excessive formation of AGE. This in turn makes you susceptible to many of today's lifestyle diseases.

So the next time you reach for that donut or that candy bar, think how much more you would age as a result of eating it.

Appendix G

Oxidation and Modern Disease

"No disease that can be treated by diet should be treated with any other means."

Maimonides

In this section, you will understand:

- The real cause for most modern age-related degenerative diseases like heart disease, diabetes, age-related dementia, and many others.

Modern medicine regards all chronic diseases to be caused by discrete causes. Heart disease is considered a disease of cholesterol malfunction. Diabetes is considered a disease of sugar malfunction, and so on and so forth. But recent evidence suggests a common link between all these modern ailments, and that is oxidative damage and the resulting inflammation. These two factors lie at the root of all modern disease. Let's see why.

Oxidation is the process whereby oxygen reacts with elements to form oxides. An example most people are familiar with is rust, or Iron oxide. The energy centers of our cells, the mitochondria, also produce a lot of oxygen as a byproduct of the energy-generating mechanism. This oxygen is highly reactive and is termed reactive oxygen species (ROS). These reactive oxygen species oxidize other healthy molecules so the molecules are not able to function as intended. For example, ROS attacks proteins and fats, making them unstable. As a result, they start behaving in unusual ways. If

ROS attacks LDL particles, it makes them "sticky" (normal LDL isn't sticky), leading to plaque formation in the long run. A ROS attack on the DNA chain causes cross-linkage that can make it mutagenic (capable of mutating into malignant cells). All of these changes inhibit proper function and health and can cause serious disease.

Apart from ROS, there are other types of oxidizing agents in the body, known as free radicals, which can come from external sources. Processed foods loaded with preservatives, artificial food coloring agents, and other chemicals can cause the buildup of free radicals in the body that, like ROS, can attack and modify other healthy molecules and cells. Some examples of external sources of free radicals are environmental pollutants, cigarette smoke, and heavy metals in polluted water. AGE radicals from excess sugar in our blood can also do the same damage.

Inflammation: A Key Driver of Modern Disease

Whenever a molecule oxidizes from a ROS attack, the body initiates an inflammatory cycle to get rid of this modified particle. Broadly speaking, inflammation is the body's immune system response to something that might turn out to be harmful. White blood cells and lymphocytes are called on to the site of attack to "eliminate" this modified particle. When a cell suffers death, it releases ROS. This signals the immune system to eliminate and recycle the cell components. ROS have even been shown to play a role in identification and elimination of cancerous cells throughout our body. Essentially, ROS signaling plays an important part in scavenging dead cells, so some amount of ROS production is actually beneficial to immunity and good health.

The body produces its own supply of endogenous antioxidants (superoxide dismutase and glutathione) that go after these reactive oxygen species and neutralize them, but the urbanization and industrialization of the developed world in the past century have increased the oxidative load to a disproportionate amount for body's own antioxidant mechanisms to suffice. This has led to an increase in oxidative damage and inflammation-related degenerative diseases.

In the following sections, you will see how this double whammy of oxidation and inflammation is a key player in the pathogenesis of most modern diseases.

Oxidative Damage and Heart Disease

In a normal healthy artery, the innermost layer is covered by a thin lining of cells called the endothelium. This lining acts as a filter for transporting material, like white blood cells, in and out of the bloodstream. The endothelial lining is also responsible for controlling the blood pressure by relaxing and contracting the artery. LDL particles, especially the small dense LDL (sdLDL), can move in and out of the endothelial lining. The problem comes when these sdLDL particles get oxidized. These altered and oxidized LDL particles (also known as ox-LDL) then start sticking together to form large drops of ox-LDL[132].

This is where inflammation comes into play. As these coalesced ox-LDL particles reach larger sizes, they start an inflammatory response by the artery to clean up and scavenge these damaged particles. White blood cells (monocytes and lymphocytes), primarily meant for fighting external pathogens, get called in to clean up these globs of ox-LDL particles. Just as a vacuum cleaner sucks up dirt and debris, these monocytes start gobbling up large quantities of ox-LDL particles. As small droplets of oil suspended in water start attracting each other to form large drops of oil, these monocytes start attracting more altered and oxidized proteins and lipids found in the tissue as they continue to grow in size. At this point, the monocytes turn into macrophages, which are the most important cleanup cells found in tissues.

Over a period of time (years to decades) the cholesterol-rich core in the macrophages keeps expanding to form a plaque, which develops a fibrous cap on top just as a scab develops when we scrape our knee on the pavement. Over time, this fibrous protective cap starts eroding from underneath as the cholesterol deposits continue and as more and more free radical damage occurs around it. Eventually, the fibrous cap becomes unstable, ruptures, and falls off, ripping the endothelial lining in the process. This causes a rapid clot formation at the site of rupture. A large enough clot will completely block off the flow of blood in the artery. This phenomenon of plaque formation and progression is shown in Figure 18.

When such a ruptured plaque clot happens in an artery that supplies blood to the heart, the person suffers a heart attack[133]. When this happens in an artery supplying blood to the brain, the person suffers an ischemic stroke[134]. Depending on how much blood supply is cut off, permanent organ damage, and paralysis or death, may result.

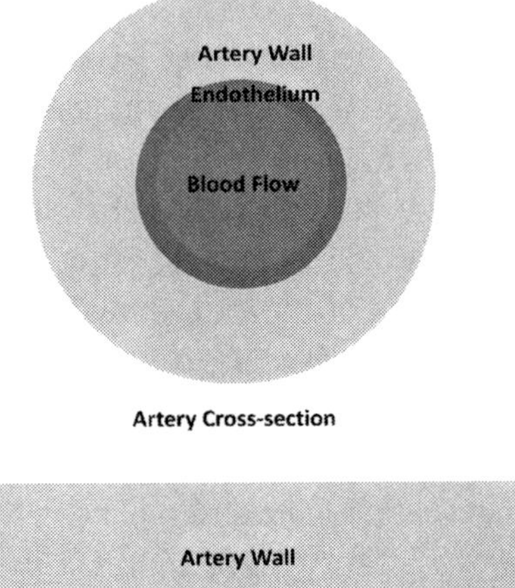

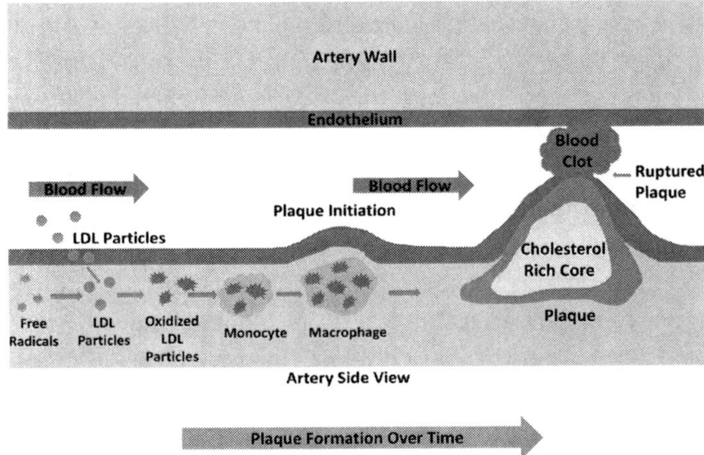

Figure 18: Schematic representation of plaque formation over time.

The bottom line is this: free radical attack in the endothelial lining initiates the formation of plaque and the resulting inflammation facilitates its growth. In fact, inflammation plays such a crucial role in the formation of plaque that markers of inflammation in the blood, also known as C-Reactive Proteins (CRP), are better predictors of heart disease than total or LDL cholesterol levels.

All the recent studies point to inflammation as being the real cause for heart disease. This is why moving away from traditional, natural sources of saturated fats like butter and red meat and replacing them with pro-inflammatory vegetable oils has only made our heart health worse in the past half-century.

Oxidation Damage and Age-related Dementia

The brain cells are metabolizing glucose at a high rate. As a result, they are a big source of local free radical production. The neuronal cells are especially prone to free radical attack because they contain a higher percentage of fatty acids, which are prone to oxidation[135]. In addition, the antioxidant activity is especially low in the brain tissue compared to other tissues around the body[136]. With age, the brain also accumulates several metals (copper, iron, and zinc) that act as a catalyst in speeding up oxidation[137].

Alzheimer's disease (AD) is caused when certain peptides react with free radicals in the presence of these metal ions to form amyloid plaques that deposit in parts of the brain[138]. Parkinson's disease (PD) is also characterized by certain deposits (Lewy bodies) in parts of the brain due to dopamine's ability to react with certain metals and generate free radicals[139].

Free radicals are also implicated in the initiation and progression of several other neurodegenerative disorders like cerebral ischemia, schizophrenia, Multiple Sclerosis (MS), and Amyotrophic Lateral Sclerosis (ALS)[140, 141, 142].

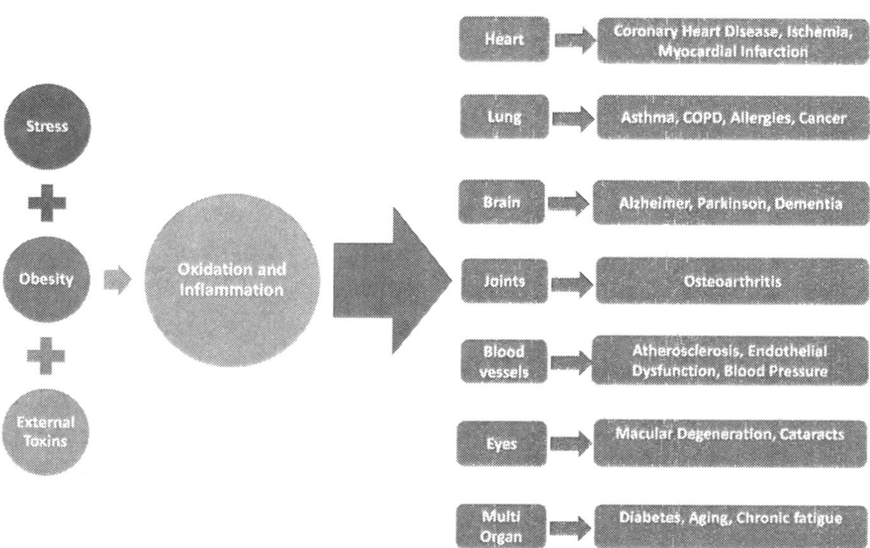

Figure 19: Oxidative damage and inflammation: cause and effect.

Cholesterol in the brain and central nervous system acts as a protective agent against oxidation. When the brain cells are starved of cholesterol due to cholesterol lowering medications (statins) it causes a rise in oxidative damage and acceleration of neurodegenerative disorders.

Free radicals can also attack the DNA strands, causing them to get cross-linked, which has been implicated in various effects of ageing, especially cancer[143]. They can attack and cause cross-linkage of fats and proteins (just as AGE do), leading to the formation of wrinkles[144].

Figure 19 shows the causes and effects of oxidation and inflammation in a snapshot. The three biggest causes of oxidative damage and inflammation are the triple assault of obesity, stress, and external toxins. The detrimental effects are visible in various organs throughout our body.

Antioxidants: The Wellness Agents

Nature has provided a lot of exogenous (external) antioxidant molecules in wholesome sources of carbohydrates in the form of vitamin A, C, E, selenium and many other polyphenols. Having antioxidant rich wholesome carbs in your diet supplements your own body's inherent supply of antioxidants in preventing oxidative damage.

The antioxidant content of foods is measured in ORAC which stands for Oxygen Radical Absorbance Capacity and measures the ability to neutralize oxygen radicals in a test tube with reactive radicals. The higher the ORAC value the higher the amount of free radicals it can neutralize, or in other words, the more potent antioxidant it is.

Although antioxidants have been found to help with weight loss, the main reason they should be a part of healthy diet is because of their value in protecting us from oxidative damage.

Studies on simple cell structures have shown age prolonging effects of antioxidants[145]. Studies on humans have shown that antioxidants may have a beneficial effect on many lifestyle and age related disorders like atherosclerosis[146, 147], cancer and some neurodegenerative[148] and ocular (like cataracts) diseases[149, 150],. This improves the quality of life as we age.

Spice: The Antioxidant Powerhouse

Spice doesn't fall strictly in the category of any macronutrient (namely fat, protein, or carbohydrate) and is regarded as a condiment or seasoning, but I put it in the carbohydrate section as it's nearer to a carbohydrate than anything else. For the small quantities used in cooking, it doesn't add any caloric value to food but offers definite medicinal and healing value.

Traditional Asian cooking uses many herbs and spices but sadly we are losing our traditional diets in favor of the more exotic fast foods perpetuated by the big food industries. In the daily hustle bustle of our busy lives, we forgo eating home cooked traditional meals and eat processed food on the run. And just to feel good about our lousy diets we will throw in a vitamin infused energy drink here and there and think that we have undone the damage.

Many ethnic dishes use turmeric, cloves, coriander, curry powder, and other traditional spices. When it comes to antioxidant content, these power-packed superfoods leave their fruit counter parts in dust. So for example the ORAC value of turmeric and cloves is 127,068 and 290,283 respectively. Compare this to the venerable Acai berry, which only has a value of 5,500. Even in its most concentrated form (pulp/skin dehydrated powder) it only has a value of 102,700 which is still 25% lesser than turmeric.

Out of all the spices studied to date, turmeric is one of the most widely studied spices in medical science. Turmeric is an herb from the ginger family and the active ingredient in it is a chemical called curcumin. Studies have shown that curcumin is a powerful anti-inflammatory and has shown to inhibit the growth of various cancerous tumors especially of the pharynx[151], breast[152] and colon[153]. Latest research suggests that curcumin also inhibits Nuclear Factor kappa B (NFkB), a chemical that binds to the DNA and is responsible for all stages of cancer initiation and growth.

Some studies have even identified it as a powerful antidepressant in the way it influences neurotransmitters such as serotonin and dopamine[154, 155]. It also has shown to be beneficial for age related neurodegenerative diseases like Parkinson's disease[156].

Cloves, cinnamon, oregano and turmeric are some of the most powerful antioxidants known to man that are used in extensively in Asian cuisine. Other Indian spices like curry powder, coriander powder, black pepper etc. are also rich in antioxidants. Appendix H lists all the food items with their ORAC values.

Cacao found in chocolate is also rich in antioxidants but most chocolate is loaded with sugar that negates any positive effect of the antioxidants. If you like chocolate, eat only an ounce per day of the bittersweet or semisweet kind that has at least 70% cacao or more.

The table below lists all the common spices along with their ORAC values (in increasing order):

Spice	ORAC	Spice	ORAC
cardamom	2,764	basil, dried	61,063
onion powder	4,289	nutmeg, ground	69,640
garlic powder	6,665	parsley, dried	73,670
pepper, red or cayenne	19,671	Szechuan pepper, dried	118,400
paprika	21,932	sage, ground	119,929
chili powder	23,636	vanilla beans, dried	122,400
mustard seed, yellow	29,257	turmeric, ground	127,068
pepper, black	34,053	cinnamon, ground	131,420
ginger, ground	39,041	thyme, dried	157,380
pepper, white	40,700	rosemary, dried	165,280
curry powder	48,504	oregano, dried	175,295
cumin seed	50,372	cloves, ground	290,283

Appendix H

Antioxidant Capacity of Common Foods

Antioxidant capacity of common foods and beverages measured in terms of Oxygen Radical Absorbance Capacity. Higher value indicates a greater ability to neutralize the effect of free radicals in the body. Arranged by decreasing antioxidant content.

Food	Oxygen Radical Absorbance Capacity
Sumac, bran, raw	312,400
Spices, cloves, ground	290,283
Sorghum, bran, hi-tannin	240,000
Spices, oregano, dried	175,295
Spices, rosemary, dried	165,280
Spices, thyme, dried	157,380
Spices, cinnamon, ground	131,420
Spices, turmeric, ground	127,068
Spices, vanilla beans, dried	122,400
Spices, sage, ground	119,929
Spices, Szechuan pepper, dried	118,400
Acai, fruit pulp/skin, powder	102,700
Sorghum, bran, black	100,800
Rosehip	96,150
Sumac, grain, raw	86,800
Spices, parsley, dried	73,670

Food	Oxygen Radical Absorbance Capacity
Sorghum, bran, red	71,000
Spices, nutmeg, ground	69,640
Spices, basil, dried	61,063
Cocoa, dry powder, unsweetened	55,653
Spices, cumin seed	50,372
Baking chocolate, unsweetened, squares	49,944
Spices, curry powder	48,504
Sorghum, grain, hi-tannin	45,400
Spices, pepper, white	40,700
Chocolate, dutched powder	40,200
Spices, ginger, ground	39,041
Spices, pepper, black	34,053
Sage, fresh	32,004
Spices, mustard seed, yellow	29,257
Thyme, fresh	27,426
Marjoram, fresh	27,297
Rice bran, crude	24,287
Spices, chili powder	23,636
Spices, paprika	21,932
Sorghum, grain, black	21,900
Candies, chocolate, dark	20,816
Spices, pepper, red or cayenne	19,671
Raspberries, black	19,220
Candies, semisweet chocolate	18,053
Nuts, pecans	17,940
Chokeberry, raw	16,062
Tarragon, fresh	15,542
Ginger root, raw	14,840
Elderberries, raw	14,697
Sorghum, grain, red	14,000
Peppermint, fresh	13,978
Oregano, fresh	13,970
Nuts, walnuts, English	13,541
Juice, black raspberry	10,460
Raisins, golden seedless	10,450
Nuts, hazelnuts or filberts	9,645
Blueberries, wild, raw	9,621

Food	Oxygen Radical Absorbance Capacity
Pears, dried to 40% moisture (purchased in Italy)	9,496
Savory, fresh	9,465
Artichokes, Ocean Mist, boiled	9,416
Artichokes, Ocean Mist, Microwaved	9,402
Cranberries, raw	9,090
Beans, kidney, red, mature seeds, raw	8,606
Beans, black, mature seeds, raw	8,494
Beans, pink, mature seeds, raw	8,320
Plums, dried (prunes), uncooked	8,059
Beans, pinto, mature seeds, raw	8,033
Currants, European black, raw	7,957
Nuts, pistachio nuts, raw	7,675
Plums, black diamond, with peel, raw	7,581
Agave, dried (Southwest)	7,524
Candies, milk chocolate	7,519
Lentils, raw	7,282
Apples, dried to 40% moisture	6,681
Spices, garlic powder	6,665
Artichokes raw	6,552
Beans, black turtle soup, mature seeds, raw	6,416
Sorghum, bran, white	6,400
Chocolate syrup	6,330
Baby food, fruit, peaches	6,257
Plums, raw	6,100
Lemon balm, leaves, raw	5,997
Blackberries, raw	5,905
Garlic, raw	5,708
Soybeans, mature seeds, raw	5,409
Coriander (cilantro) leaves, raw	5,141
Raspberries, raw	5,065
Baby food, fruit, apple and blueberry, junior	4,822
Basil, fresh	4,805
Blueberries, raw	4,669
Alcoholic beverage wine, table, red, Cabernet Sauvignon	4,523
Pomegranates, raw	4,479
Nuts, almonds	4,454

Food	Oxygen Radical Absorbance Capacity
Dill weed, fresh	4,392
Cowpeas, common (blackeyes, crowder, southern), mature seeds, raw	4,343
Strawberries, raw	4,302
Spices, onion powder	4,289
Apples, Red Delicious, raw. with skin	4,275
Peaches, dried to 40% moisture	4,222
Raisins, white, dried to 40% moisture	4,188
Baby food, fruit, applesauce, strained	4,123
Apples, Granny Smith, raw, with skin	3,898
Dates, deglet noor	3,895
Cherries, sweet, raw	3,747
Makiang, raw	3,695
Alcoholic beverage, wine, table, red	3,607
Peanut butter, smooth style	3,432
Raisins, seedless	3,406
Currants, red, raw	3,387
Figs, raw	3,383
Gooseberries, raw	3,332
Goji berry (wolfberry), raw	3,290
Apricots, dried to 40% moisture (purchased in Italy)	3,234
Peanuts, all types, raw	3,166
Cabbage, red, boiled	3,145
Broccoli raab, raw	3,083
Agave, cooked (Southwest)	3,074
Apples, raw, with skin	3,049
Apples, Red Delicious, raw, without skin	2,936
Apples, Gala, raw, with skin	2,828
Spices, cardamom	2,764
Pomegranate juice, bottled	2,681
Alcoholic Beverage, wine, table, red, Merlot	2,670
Apples, Golden Delicious, raw, with skin	2,670
Baby food, fruit, bananas	2,658
Maloud, raw	2,611
Apples, Fuji, raw, with skin	2,589
Apples, raw, without skin	2,573
Baby food, fruit, peaches, junior	2,551

Food	Oxygen Radical Absorbance Capacity
Guava, white-fleshed	2,550
Mangosteen, raw	2,510
Cabbage, red, raw	2,496
Lettuce, red leaf, raw	2,426
Alcoholic Beverage, wine, table, red, Zinfandel	2,400
Juice, Concord grape	2,389
Dates, medjool	2,387
Juice, black cherry	2,370
Cereals, ready-to-eat, corn flakes	2,359
Juice, Blueberry	2,359
Cereals, oats, instant, fortified, plain, dry	2,308
Cereals ready-to-eat, granola, low-fat, with raisins	2,294
Asparagus, raw	2,252
Beans, black, mature seeds, boiled	2,249
Apples, Golden Delicious, raw, without skin	2,210
Cauliflower, purple, cooked	2,210
Pears, green cultivars, with peel, raw	2,201
Sorghum, grain, white	2,200
Radish seeds, sprouted, raw	2,184
Cereals ready-to-eat, oat bran	2,183
Cereals ready-to-eat, toasted oatmeal	2,175
Cereals, oats, quick, uncooked	2,169
Broccoli, boiled	2,160
Cereals ready-to-eat, oatmeal, toasted squares	2,143
Sweet potato, baked in skin	2,115
Bread, butternut whole grain	2,104
Oranges, raw, all commercial varieties	2,103
Chives, raw	2,094
Cauliflower, purple, raw	2,084
Cabbage, savoy, boiled	2,050
Prune juice, canned	2,036
Guava, red-fleshed	1,990
Applesauce, canned, unsweetened, without added ascorbic acid	1,965
Bread, pumpernickel	1,963
Nuts, cashew nuts, raw	1,948
Beet greens, raw	1,946

Food	Oxygen Radical Absorbance Capacity
Avocados, Hass, raw	1,922
Peaches, raw	1,922
Arugula (rocket), raw	1,904
Beans, navy, mature seeds, raw	1,861
Snacks, tortilla chips, low fat, made with olestra, nacho cheese	1,858
Grapes, red, raw	1,837
Oranges, raw, navels	1,819
Juice, red grape	1,788
Beets, raw	1,776
Cabbage, black, cooked	1,773
Juice, acai blends	1,767
Radishes, raw	1,750
Grapes, black	1,746
Pears, red Anjou, raw	1,746
Snacks, popcorn, air-popped	1,743
Cereals, oats, old fashioned, uncooked	1,708
Nuts, macadamia nuts, dry roasted	1,695
Spinach, frozen, chopped or leaf, unprepared	1,687
Potatoes, Russet, flesh and skin, baked	1,680
Asparagus, cooked, boiled, drained	1,644
Grapefruit, raw, pink and red and white, all areas	1,640
Tangerines, (mandarin oranges), raw	1,627
Broccoli raab, cooked	1,590
Snacks, tortilla chips, low fat, made with olestra	1,549
Grapefruit, raw, pink and red, all areas	1,548
Lettuce, green leaf, raw	1,532
Onions, red, raw	1,521
Spinach, raw	1,513
Alfalfa seeds, sprouted, raw	1,510
Broccoli, raw	1,510
Juice, Cranberry/Concord grape	1,480
Cranberry juice, unsweetened	1,452
Lettuce, butterhead raw	1,423
Guavas, common, raw	1,422
Bread, Multi-Grain (includes whole-grain)	1,421
Nuts, brazil nuts, dried, unblanched	1,419

Food.......	Oxygen Radical Absorbance Capacity
Cauliflower, green, cooked	1,387
Lemons, raw, without peel	1,346
Potatoes, red, flesh and skin, baked	1,326
Potatoes, russet, flesh and skin, raw	1,322
Bread, Oatnut	1,318
Cereals ready-to-eat, wheat, shredded, plain, sugar and salt free	1,303
Parsley, raw	1,301
Mangos, raw	1,300
Agave, raw (Southwest)	1,294
Milk, chocolate, fluid, commercial, reduced fat	1,263
Tea, green, brewed	1,253
Grapefruit juice, white, raw	1,238
Lemon juice, raw	1,225
Onions, yellow, sautéed	1,220
Kiwi, gold, raw	1,210
Potatoes, white, flesh and skin, baked	1,138
Tea, brewed, prepared with tap water	1,128
Apricots, raw	1,110
Potatoes, red, flesh and skin, raw	1,098
Potatoes, white, flesh and skin, raw	1,058
Peppers, sweet, yellow, raw	1,043
Grapes, white or green, raw	1,018
Lettuce, cos or romaine, raw	1,017
Alcoholic beverage, wine, table, rose	1,005
Juice, strawberry	1,002
Sauce, salsa, ready-to-serve	1,001
Peppers, sweet, orange, raw	984
Mushrooms, portabella, raw	968
Soybeans, mature seeds, sprouted, raw	962
Mushrooms, brown, Italian, or Crimini, raw	951
Pineapple, raw, extra sweet variety	943
Peppers, sweet, green, raw	935
Eggplant, raw	932
Nectarines, raw	919
Onions, raw	913
Beans, pinto, mature seeds, boiled	904

Food	Oxygen Radical Absorbance Capacity
Sweet potato, raw	902
Cauliflower, raw	870
Juice, Cranberry, 100% - cranberry blend, red	865
Onions, white, raw	863
Kiwi fruit, (Chinese gooseberries), fresh, raw	862
Cabbage, boiled	856
Chickpeas (garbanzo beans, Bengal gram), mature seeds, raw	847
Peppers, sweet, red, sautéed	847
Lime juice, raw	823
Peppers, sweet, red, raw	821
Noni fruit, raw	800
Beans, snap, green, raw	799
Bananas, raw	795
Juice, white grape	793
Olive oil, extra-virgin, w/parsley, home prepared	766
Sweet potato, cooked, boiled, without skin	766
Mushrooms, shiitake, dried	752
Peas, yellow, mature seeds, raw	741
Chilchen (Red Berry Beverage) (Navajo)	740
Cauliflower, boiled	739
Corn, sweet, yellow, raw	728
Orange juice, raw	726
Nuts, pine nuts, dried	720
Pear juice, all varieties	704
Orange juice, canned, unsweetened	703
Carrots, raw	697
Peppers, sweet, yellow, grilled	694
Tomato products, canned, sauce	694
Mushrooms, white, raw	691
Mush, blue corn with ash (Navajo)	684
Olive oil, extra-virgin, w/basil, home prepared	684
Mushrooms, maitake, raw	669
Mushroom, oyster, raw	664
Cauliflower, frozen, unprepared	620
Peppers, sweet, green, sautéed	615
Onions, sweet, raw	614

Food. . . . . . Oxygen Radical Absorbance Capacity

Peas, green, frozen, unprepared 600
Syrups, maple 590
Catsup 578
Leeks, (bulb and lower leaf-portion), raw 569
Pineapple juice, canned, unsweetened, without added ascorbic acid 568
Vinegar, Apple 564
Pineapple, raw, traditional varieties 562
Olive oil, extra-virgin, w/garlic, home prepared. 557
Celery, raw. 552
Vegetable juice cocktail, canned. .548
Tomatoes, plum, raw 546
Cabbage, raw. 529
Peas, split, mature seeds, raw 524
Corn, sweet, yellow, frozen, kernels cut off cob, unprepared 522
Tea, green, ready-to-drink 520
Broccoli, frozen, spears, unprepared 496
Tomato juice, canned 486
Cocoa mix, powder. 485
Pumpkin, raw. 483
Spices, poppy seed 481
Lettuce, iceberg (includes crisphead types), raw 438
Carrots, baby, raw. 436
Peaches, canned, heavy syrup, drained 436
Tomatoes, red, ripe, cooked 423
Apple juice, canned or bottled, unsweetened, without added ascorbic acid 414
Baby food, juice, pear. 414
Corn, sweet, yellow, canned, brine pack, regular pack, solids and liquids 413
Vinegar, Red wine 410
Squash, winter, butternut, raw 396
Alcoholic beverage, wine, table, white 392
Tomatoes, red, ripe, raw, year round average 387
Pineapple, raw, all varieties 385
Olive oil, extra-virgin 372

Food. . . . . . Oxygen Radical Absorbance Capacity

Carrots, boiled. 326

Melons, cantaloupe, raw 319

Tea, black, ready-to-drink, plain and flavored 313

Fennel, bulb, raw 307

Papayas, raw 300

Asparagus, white, raw. 296

Beans, snap, green variety, canned, regular pack, solids and liquids. 290

Vinegar, Apple and Honey 270

Tea, white, ready-to-drink 264

Banana, Nam-wa variety. 260

Melons, honeydew, raw 253

Eggplant, boiled 245

Beans, lima, immature seeds, canned, regular pack, solids and liquids 243

Cucumber, with peel, raw. 232

Juice, Cranberry, white. 232

Vinegar, Honey 225

Olive oil, extra-virgin, w/garlic and red hot peppers, home prepared 219

Squash, summer, zucchini, includes skin, raw 180

Watermelon, raw. 142

Cucumber, peeled, raw. 140

Cauliflower, green, raw 136

Oil, peanut, salad or cooking. 106

Limes, raw 82

Suggested Further References

Fat doesn't make you fat, Processed carbs and sugar do

- *Fat Chance: Beating the Odds Against Sugar, Processed Food, Obesity, and Disease*, by Robert H. Lustig, Hudson Street Press, 2013.
- *Pure, White, and Deadly: How Sugar Is Killing Us and What We Can Do to Stop It*, by John Yudkin and Robert H. Lustig, Penguin Books, 2013.
- *Good Calories, Bad Calories: Fats, Carbs, and the Controversial Science of Diet and Health*, by Gary Taubes, First Anchor Books, 2008.
- *Why we get fat and what to do about it*, by Gary Taubes, published by Alfred A Knopf, a division of Random House Inc., 2011.
- *Wheat Belly; Lose the Wheat, Lose the Weight, and Find Your Path Back to Health*, by William Davis, MD., Rodale Books, 2011.
- *Grain Brain: The Surprising Truth about Wheat, Carbs, and Sugar—Your Brain's Silent Killers*, by David Perlmutter and Kristin Loberg, Little, Brown and Company, 2013.

Understanding Fat Metabolism

- www.westonaprice.org/know-your-fats/ (Weston Price Foundation)
- *Eat Fat, Lose Fat: The Healthy Alternative to Trans Fats*, by Mary Enig and Sally Fallon, Hudson Street Press (Penguin Group), 2006.

- *Nourishing Traditions: The Cookbook that Challenges Politically Correct Nutrition and the Diet Dictocrats* by Sally Fallon and Mary Enig, New Trends Publishing, 2012.

Cholesterol and Saturated Fat are good for you (and they don't cause heart disease)

- *The Big Fat Surprise: Why Butter, Meat and Cheese Belong in a Healthy Diet*, by Nina Teicholz, Simon and Schuster, 2014.

- *The Great Cholesterol Con: The Truth About What Really Causes Heart Disease and How to Avoid It*, by Malcolm Kendrick, John Blake Publishing Ltd, 2008.

- *Ignore the Awkward: How the Cholesterol Myths Are Kept Alive*, by Uffe Ravnskov, 2010.

- *Fat and Cholesterol are Good for You*, by Uffe Ravnskov, GB Publishing, 2009.

- *The Cholesterol Myths: Exposing the Fallacy that Saturated Fat and Cholesterol Cause Heart Disease*, By Uffe Ravnskov, 2000.

Inflammation and Chronic Disease Prevention

- *Advanced Nutrition; Macronutrients, Micronutrients, and Metabolism*, Carolyn D. B., Janos Z., CRC Press, 2009.

- *The Anti-Inflammation Zone: Reversing the Silent Epidemic That's Destroying Our Health*, by Barry Sears, HarperCollins, 2005.

- *Inflammation Nation: The First Clinically Proven Eating Plan to End Our Nation's Secret Epidemic*, by Ph.D. Floyd H. Chilton Ph.D. and Laura Tucker, Fireside (a registered trademark of Simon and Schuster), 2006.

The Role of Omega-3 Fats in Human Health

- *Omega-6/Omega-3 Essential Fatty Acid Ratio: The Scientific Evidence (World Review of Nutrition and Dietetics, Vol. 92)*, by A.P. Simopoulos (Editor), L.G. Cleland (Editor), B. Koletzko (Series Editor), Karger, 2003.

- *The Omega-3 Effect: Everything You Need to Know About the Supernutrient for Living Longer, Happier, and Healthier*, by William Sears and James Sears, Little, Brown and Company, 2012.

- *The Omega Diet: The Lifesaving Nutritional Program Based on the Diet of the Island of Crete*, by Artemis P. Simopoulos and Jo Robinson, Harper Collins, 1998.

Nutrition for Weight Loss and Wellness

- *Always Hungry? Conquer Cravings, Retrain Your Fat Cells, and Lose Weight Permanently*, by David Ludwig Hachette Group, 2016.

- *The Blood Sugar Solution: The Ultra Healthy Program for Losing Weight, Preventing Disease, and Feeling Great Now*, by Mark Hyman, Little, Brown and Company, 2012.

Eating Organic Resources

- http://www.eatwild.com/

- http://farmersmarketcoalition.org/networking/state-associations/

- https://www.organicconsumers.org/organlink

Glossary And Terms

Adipoinsular axis: A feedback system between the two hormones, insulin and leptin, that strives to maintain energy stores in the body to a tightly regulated set-point. In a healthy body this prevents overeating and starvation.

Adipose tissue: Scientific name for fat tissue.

Advanced Glycation End-product (AGE): As the name suggests these molecules (or end products) are formed when glucose reacts with (or glycates) lipids and proteins. AGE formation is known to speed up oxidation and is causally linked to many chronic degenerative disorders related to diabetes

Alzheimer's: A chronic degenerative disease of the brain whereby the patient loses his memory and slowly as the disease progresses, further loses his orientation, motivation and develops behavioral issues

Atherosclerosis: A disease of the arteries that is characterized by plaque deposits on the walls of the arteries.

Basal Metabolic Rate (BMR): The amount of energy burned by the body at rest. Also known as resting metabolic rate (RMR). This is the minimum amount of energy required by the body to sustain the function of all the vital organs.

Body Mass Index (BMI): An obesity metric that is derived by dividing the bodyweight by the square of the body height expressed in the units of KG/m^2.

Calorie: A unit of energy. A food calorie is the amount of energy required to heat a kilogram of water by one degree Celsius. Also represented as kilocalorie in some labels.

Carbohydrates: A macronutrient component in diet that primarily consists of long chains of sugar molecules. Gets broken down in the gut into small sugar molecules to be absorbed in the blood and provide energy to the cells throughout the body.

Chemoattractant Protein: A molecule that attracts immune cells to the sites of inflammation that occur either from tissue injury or infection.

Cholesterol: A waxy substance that's synthesized in the human body and is incorporated in the cell membranes to provide structural rigidity and protection from external environment. Also used in the production of all the sex hormones and bile acids for digestion.

C-Reactive Protein (CRP): A protein molecule that is synthesized in the liver. The levels of CRP are proportional to the level of inflammation in the body.

Diabetes Mellitus: Scientific name for Diabetes, which is marked by the inability of the pancreas to make insulin.

Docosahexaenoic acid (DHA): belongs to the omega-3 class of essential fats and is primarily used in the formation of the human brain, cerebral cortex, skin, sperms, testicles and retina. The human body doesn't make any DHA and it has to come from dietary sources.

Eicosanoids: These are super hormones that are formed at the point of use by every cell and their primary role is to act as a signaling molecule to determine the action of hormones on those cells.

Eicosapentaenoic acid (EPA): is a polyunsaturated fat that is the precursor to the formation of eicosanoids. It belongs to the omega-3 class of fatty acids. EPA is an essential fat that's needed in the diet, as it cannot be synthesized in the body.

Estrogen: The female sex hormone that is responsible for sexual development and the female reproductive system.

Fatty Acids: A fatty acid is a carboxylic acid attached to a long chain of carbons and hydrogens. Most FAs have an unbranched carbon-carbon chain of varying length. Based on the length of the carbon chain they are further subdivided into short, medium, long and very long chain fatty acids.

Free Radical: A molecule that's lacking a paired electron in the outermost (valence) shell. Electrons like to be paired, which makes these unpaired electron molecules highly reactive. Free radicals spontaneously attack other molecules around them to satisfy their need for pairing this outermost electron.

Free Range: A term used to describe animal farming practice where the animals (or birds) are left in the wild to forage on their natural diet. This has been shown to produce meat with a higher nutritional value and has the ideal omega-6/omega-3 ratio and has lowered levels of stress hormones.

Gastric Bypass Surgery: A surgical procedure where the stomach is divided into two parts and the small intestine is then connected to both parts of the stomach. This effectively reduces the functional volume of the stomach there by reducing appetite and the physical response to food. It is used as a treatment method for morbid obesity.

Ghee: Clarified butter fat. Popular in Indian cuisine

Ghrelin: The main "hunger" hormone that is produced in the stomach when it's empty. It regulates the appetite by increasing hunger and by preparing the stomach for incoming food. Once the stomach is stretched, its production ceases.

Glycemic Index: A relative measure of how fast a given food raises blood sugar level. The comparison baseline is that of pure glucose which is assigned an arbitrary value of 100.

Glycogen: A type of sugar molecule that's made in the liver from dietary carbohydrates. It is the main form of energy storage in cells for short-term use in the body.

GMO: Stands for Genetically Modified Organism and is any organism whose genetic material has been restructured using genetic engineering techniques. It's commonly being used to create crops that are resistant to certain pests and certain environmental conditions.

HbA1C: is another name for glycated hemoglobin, the main oxygen-carrying protein molecule in the blood. HbA1C is measured to determine average blood glucose levels over prolonged periods of time (typically 3 months). It reveals more about a person's diet and lifestyle than fasting glucose test.

HDL: an acronym that stands for high density lipoprotein. It's a carrier molecule that is used to transport fat and cholesterol from the point of use back to the liver for recycling. It is also referred to as "good" cholesterol.

HFCS: an acronym for High Fructose Corn Syrup, a corn-derived sweetener that's predominantly used in many soft drinks and beverages in place of table sugar.

Homeostasis: A system property that keeps variables regulated in a small range of control, for example maintaining the body temperature or pH of blood. This is a way for nature to maintain life-sustaining conditions in control.

Hypothalamus: The portion of the brain that controls metabolic and homeostatic processes in the body like sleep, hunger, thirst and body temperature. It also links the nervous system to the endocrine system via the pituitary gland forming what is typically referred to as the Hypothalamic-Pituitary-Adrenal axis (HPA axis). The HPA axis regulates many of the vital body functions like reactions to stress, mood and emotions, sexuality, energy storage and expenditure, digestion, and immunity.

Inflammation: A biological response of the body tissue to harmful stimuli such has invading pathogens, injury, or other toxins.

Insulin: The main storage hormone synthesized on the beta cells of pancreas that is involved in the sugar and fat metabolism.

Interleukin: special proteins and signaling molecules that are expressed by while blood cells and play an important role in immunity.

lbLDL: This is a type of Low Density Lipoprotein, a molecule that transports cholesterol to the site of use, that is classified based on its size and buoyancy. This type of LDL is large and more buoyant than its smaller and denser LDL cousin also known as sdLDL. Saturated fat is known to increase the production of lbLDL. lbLDL is resistant to oxidation and is NOT implicated in the formation of plaque.

LDL: an acronym that stands for Low Density Lipoprotein. It's a carrier molecule that is used to transport fat and cholesterol to the point of use in cells and tissues. It is also referred to as "bad" cholesterol.

Leptin: The main "satiety" hormone that is responsible for maintaining long-term energy balance in the body. Leptin determines that amount of stored body fat. The hormone is produced in the adipose (fat) tissue and acts on the receptors in the Hypothalamus to regulate hunger and metabolism to maintain energy balance.

Lipid: naturally occurring molecules that include fats, sterols (like cholesterol), waxes, and fat-soluble vitamins.

Lipohypertrophy: Literally means increase in fat mass. It is fat accumulation under the skin usually at the site of insulin injections.

Macrophage: A type of white blood cell that engulfs and digests cellular debris, foreign pathogens, cancer cells or any other foreign body that has a structure different from a healthy cell. Plays an important role in immunity.

Metabolic Syndrome: A metabolic disorder where insulin resistance causes the pancreas to release large quantities of insulin to counteract elevated blood sugar but due to the insulin resistance the blood sugar level remains high. This condition is marked by abdominal obesity, increased plasma triglycerides, increased lethargy, increased thirst and urination. Usually a precursor to type II Diabetes.

Metabolism: The rate at with body burns energy. Metabolism also determines our activity level.

Mitochondria: The part of cell that produces energy.

MRI: Magnetic Resonance Imaging, a technique for imaging soft tissue as opposed to X-Rays that are used to image bones.

Nucleus Accumbens: The part of the brain responsible for motivation, reward, aversion, pleasure and reinforced learning.

ORAC: stands for Oxygen Radical Absorbance Capacity; a quantitative measure of the capability of a certain food to neutralizing reactive oxygen species and other free radicals

Oxidation: A reaction with oxygen to form oxides. For example, oxygen reacts with iron to form iron oxide (rust). A similar reaction happens in the body when reactive oxygen species react with healthy molecules (lipids, proteins, DNA etc.) to form oxidized molecules that no longer function as intended.

Ox-LDL: An oxidized LDL molecule. Ox-LDL has a tendency to stick to other Ox-LDL molecules making it the prime candidate in the formation and growth of plaque.

Parkinson's: A degenerative disease of the central nervous system that affects motor skills including shaking, difficulty moving. As the disease progresses it could lead to behavioral issues, depression, and dementia.

pH: A measure of acidity and alkalinity.

Phytoestrogens: are plant-derived estrogen-like compounds that interfere with normal estrogen function in the human body.

Protein: A Macronutrient component containing amino acids. It is also the building block of all tissues and enzymes in the body. It is involved in many important cellular functions like metabolic reaction and DNA replication.

Reactive Oxygen Species (ROS): These are chemically reactive molecules containing oxygen. ROS are formed as a natural byproduct of energy producing (oxygen) metabolism in the cell mitochondria (energy centers of the cell) and play an important role in cell signaling. However, in times of environmental stress ROS production is greatly exacerbated causing cell damage and other oxidative damage.

Resistin: A hormone that is secreted in the visceral fat cells that causes an increase in inflammation. It further increases the production of LDL (bad cholesterol) and impairs the ability of the liver to clear LDL from the body, thereby accelerating the accumulation of LDL in the arteries.

Resting Metabolic Rate (RMR): This is the minimum amount of energy burned daily to sustain vital life functions. Also known as Basal Metabolic Rate (BMR).

sdLDL: LDL is further subdivided into small dense LDL (sdLDL) which is smaller, denser and more prone to oxidation damage and primarily responsible for plaque formation in the arteries. Carbohydrates are known to increase the production of sdLDL in the body.

Statins: A class of drugs that inhibit the production of cholesterol in the body.

Subcutaneous fat: the fat immediately beneath the skin as opposed to the deeper fat surrounding the vital organs (visceral fat).

Syndrome X: another name for Metabolic Syndrome.

Testosterone: The male sex hormone that is responsible for sexual development and the male reproductive system.

Triglycerides: A molecule consisting of three fat molecules attached to a glycerol molecule to enable its transport via blood circulation. It is the main constituent of body fat in humans.

Tumor Necrosis Factor: A special protein molecule that can cause cell death.

Fasting blood sugar: the levels of blood sugar after not consuming any calories for at least 12 hours. Usually measured first thing in the morning before breakfast.

Type II Diabetes: Also known as adult onset of Diabetes. Was fairly typical for elderly populations to develop diabetes beyond a certain age but since kids in their early years started developing this type of diabetes, the name has been changed to type II Diabetes.

Visceral Fat: The deeper layers of fat surrounding the vital organs. This type of fat is associated with systemic inflammation and has been implicated in many chronic diseases.

Meet The Author

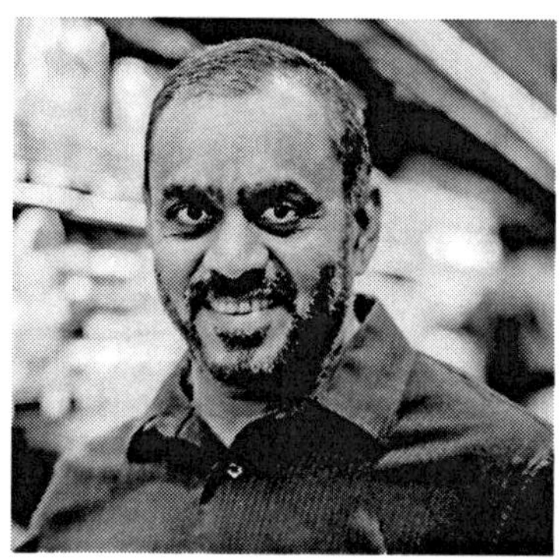

Yogesh Verma had a great interest in being healthy beginning in his teens. Growing up in the 70s and 80s during the peak of the low-fat diet era, he was strongly influenced by its supposed merits. He was mostly a vegetarian during that time, with occasional meat meals here and there.

He considered himself pretty healthy and thought he was disease-proof until he turned 26, when reality hit him: his medical reports showed high cholesterol, high triglycerides, and a high fasting sugar level. The doctor prescribed statins and the low-fat diet he was already on!

That's when he decided it was time to change things. But change to what? He was already doing everything by the book and yet there he was at the crossroads facing heart disease, diabetes, and everything else that came with them. He had no clue what he was supposed to do. He was baffled!

He continued with an even stricter version of the "healthy low-fat diet" in order to reverse his condition. He started exercising avidly, but the weight kept piling on. Four years later, and over forty pounds heavier, his health got worse.

After the birth of his first child, he decided that whatever he was doing wasn't working. It was time for a paradigm shift!

He decided to do his own research. He devoured scientific literature hoping to find the answer. In doing so, he not only discovered that he had been doing it all wrong all these years but also that the very foundation of the prescribed "low-fat healthy diet" was built on shaky grounds. He found that the science behind the low-fat diet was sparse to non-existent, and that this so-called "healthy diet" was causing more widespread harm than good.

He made drastic changes to his diet and his health improved. Soon afterward, he started blogging at inutrifit.com about healthy eating and exercising. Later on, at the urging of close friends, he started writing this book. He published several articles on nutrition for disease prevention in local magazines and periodicals such as *Siliconeer*, *Khabar*, and *India West*. He was also a featured health expert on local Bay Area radio talk shows on KLOK 1170 AM. He now hosts free seminars at public libraries and local meetup groups about healthy nutrition for weight loss and chronic disease prevention.

In 2015, he found Axiom Nutrifit, Inc., a wellness company providing weight loss and wellness solutions to individual and corporate clients. He works with clients all over the world and helps them achieve a higher state of wellness through nutrition and lifestyle counseling.

In his day job, Yogesh is a physicist working on cutting edge fuel cell technology and other renewable energy sources. In previous positions, he has contributed to the development and fabrication of world class ultra-precision fusion optics used in the National Ignition Facility at the Lawrence Livermore National Laboratory and X-Ray Synchrotron grating mirrors for the National Synchrotron Light Source at the Brookhaven National Laboratory. He has worked on many other high technology areas relating to semiconductors, photovoltaics, and high energy physics. He has published several technical papers in conferences and symposiums related to his work as a physicist.

Yogesh lives in the Bay Area with his wife and two children. When he is not writing or researching, he loves cooking, hiking, watching movies, and spending time with his friends and family. He is also an audiophile and loves building his own electron tube audio gear.

Visit www.SkinnyWithoutWillpower.com for more info.

Index

A

B

C

D

E

F

G

H

I

J

K

L

M

N

O

P

Q

R

S

T

U

V

W

Y

Z

Bibliography

Introduction

1. http://fnic.nal.usda.gov/dietary-guidance/dietary-reference-intakes/dri-tables.

Chapter 2

2. Robertson MD, Henderson RA, Vist GE, Rumsey RDE. "Extended effects of evening meal carbohydrate-to-fat ratio on fasting and postprandial substrate metabolism." *American Journal of Clinical Nutrition* 75: 505-510, 2002.

3. Luigi L., Sebastio P., Angelo C., Annalisa N., Anna L., Francesca D.S., Marilena C., Michele D. F., Vincenzo M., Vincenzo N., Mauro C., Riccardo G. and Francesco G. "Insulin Signaling in Human Visceral and Subcutaneous Adipose Tissue In Vivo." *Diabetes* vol. 55 no. 4 952-961. April 2006.

4. Reaven GM. "The metabolic syndrome: requiescat in pace." *Clinical Chemistry* 51:931-8. 2005.

5. Reaven GM. "Role of Insulin resistance in human disease. Banting lecture." *Diabetes* ;37:1595-607. 1988.

6. Best, C. H., and Scott, D. A. "The Discovery of Insulin: the Work of Frederick Banting and Charles Best." *Journal of Biological Chemistry*. 1923, 57, 709 -723.

7. Joslin's Diabetes Mellitus: Edited by C. Ronald Kahn Elliott Proctor Joslin, C. Ronald Kahn., *Lippincott Williams & Wilkins*, 2005.

8. Ludwig D.S., Majzoub J.A., Al-Zahrani A., Dallal G.E., Blanco I., Roberts S.B. "High glycemic index foods, overeating, and obesity." *Pediatrics*. 1999 Mar;103(3):E26.

9. Belinda S Lennerz, David C Alsop, Laura M Holsen, Emily Stern, Rafael Rojas, Cara B Ebbeling, Jill M Goldstein, and David S Ludwig. “Effects of dietary glycemic index on brain regions related to reward and craving in men.” *American Journal of Clinical Nutrition*, September 2013.

10. Luigi Fontana, J. Christopher Eagon, Maria E. Trujillo, Philipp E. Scherer and Samuel Klein. “Visceral Fat Adipokine Secretion Is Associated With Systemic Inflammation in Obese Humans.” *Diabetes*. April 2007 vol. 56 no. 4 1010-1013.

11. Holmes C., Cunningham C., Zotova E., Woolford J., Dean C., Kerr S., Culliford D. and Perry V. H. “Systemic inflammation and disease progression in Alzheimer disease.” *Neurology* September 8, 2009 vol. 73 no. 10 768-774.

12. Perry V. H. “The influence of systemic inflammation on inflammation in the brain: implications for chronic neurodegenerative disease.” *Brain, Behavior, and Immunity* Volume 18, Issue 5, September 2004, Pages 407–413.

13. Schapira DV1, Clark RA, Wolff PA, Jarrett AR, Kumar NB, Aziz NM. “Visceral obesity and breast cancer risk.” *Cancer*. 1994 Jul 15;74(2):632-9.

Chapter 3

14. Friedman JM. “A tale of two hormones.” *Nature Medicine*. 2010;16(10):1100–1106.

15. Friedman JM. “Modern science versus the stigma of obesity.” *Nature Medicine*. 2004; 10(6):563–569.

16. Kieffer TJ, Habener JF. “Adipoinsular axis: effects of Leptin on pancreatic beta-cells.” *American Journal of Physiology Endocrinology and Metabolism*. 2000 Jan; 278(1):E1-E14.

17. Wabitsch M, Jensen PB, Blum WF, Christoffersen CT, Englaro P, Heinze E, Rascher W, Teller W, Tornqvist H, Hauner H. “Insulin and cortisol promote Leptin production in cultured human fat cells.” *Diabetes*. 1996 Oct; 45(10):1435-8.

18. Zhao AZ, Bornfeldt KE, Beavo JA. “Leptin inhibits Insulin secretion by activation of phosphodiesterase 3B.” *Journal of Clinical Investigation*. 1998 Sep 1;102(5):869-73.

19. Ludwig DS, Friedman MI. “Increasing Adiposity, Consequence or Cause of Overeating?” *The Journal of American Medical Association*, June 4, 2014 Vol 311 number 21, 2167.

Chapter 4

20. Otsuka R, Yatsuya H, Tamakoshi K, Matsushita K, Wada K, Toyoshima H. "Perceived psychological stress and serum Leptin concentrations in Japanese men." *Obesity*, October 2006, 14 (10): 1832–1838.

21. Epel, E.S., B. McEwen, T. Seeman, et al. "Stress and body shape: stress-induced cortisol secretion is consistently greater among women with central fat." *Psychosomatic Medicine* 62:623-632, 2000.

22. Farah H., Mark A., Barbara L. C., Kristin B., Curtis B., Diane A., Eeshara K. V. "Prevalence of War-Related Mental Health Conditions and Association With Displacement Status in Postwar Jaffna District, Sri Lanka." *Journal of American Medical Association*. 2011;306(5):522-531.

23. Klatsky AL, Tekawa I, Armstrong MA, Sidney S. "The risk of hospitalization for ischemic heart disease among Asian Americans in northern California." *American Journal of Public Health*. Oct 1994;84(10):1672-1675.

24. Marmot MG, Syme SL, Kagan A, Kato H, Cohen JB, Belsky J. "Epidemiologic studies of coronary heart disease and stroke in Japanese men living in Japan, Hawaii and California: prevalence of coronary and hypertensive heart disease and associated risk factors." *American Journal of Epidemiology*. 1975 Dec;102(6):514-25.

25. K Hughes, P P Yeo, K C Lun, A C Thai, S P Sothy, K W Wang, J S Cheah, W O Phoon, P Lim. "Cardiovascular diseases in Chinese, Malays, and Indians in Singapore. II. Differences in risk factor levels." *Journal of Epidemiology and Community Health* 1990;44:29-35.

26. Dassanayake J1, Gurrin L, Payne WR, Sundararajan V, Dharmage SC. "Cardiovascular disease risk in immigrants: what is the evidence and where are the gaps?" *Asia-Pacific Journal of Public Health*. 2011 Nov;23(6):882-95.

27. Dassanayake J1, Dharmage SC, Gurrin L, Sundararajan V, Payne WR. "Are immigrants at risk of heart disease in Australia? A systematic review." *Australian Health Review*. Aug 2009;33(3):479-91.

28. Bhatnagar D, Anand I, Durrington P, Patel D, Wander G, Mackness M, Creed F, Tomenson B, Chandrashekhar Y, Winterbotham M, Britt R, Keil J & Sutton G. "Coronary risk factors in people from the Indian subcontinent living in West London and their siblings in India." *Lancet*, 1995 345, 405–409.

29. P M McKeigue, M G Marmot, Y D Syndercombe Court, D E Cottier, S Rahman, and R A Riemersma. "Diabetes, hyperinsulinemia, and coronary risk factors in Bangladeshis in east London." *British Heart Journal*. Nov 1988; 60(5): 390–396.

30. Leal-Cerro A1, Soto A, Martínez MA, Dieguez C, Casanueva FF. "Influence of cortisol status on leptin secretion." *Pituitary*. 2001 Jan-Apr;4(1-2):111-6.

31. Richard D, Barkaboi D. "Circuitries involved in the control of energy homeostasis and the hypothalamic-pituitary-adrenal axis activity." *Treat Endocrinol* 2004;3:269–77.

32. Epel E, Lapidus R, McEwen B, Brownell K. "Stress may add bite to appetite in women: a laboratory study of stress-induced cortisol and eating behavior." *Psychoneuroendocrinology* 2001;26:37–49.

33. Schellekens H, Finger BC, Dinan TG, Cryan JF. "Ghrelin signalling and obesity: at the interface of stress, mood and food reward." *Pharmacology & Therapeutics*. 2012 Sep;135(3):316-26.

34. Fernstrom JD, Wurtman RJ. "Brain Serotonin Content: Physiological Regulation by Plasma Neutral Amino Acids." *Obesity Research* Volume 5, Issue 4, 6 SEP 2012.

35. Jane E. Brody. "How Diet Can Affect Mood and Behavior" *The New York Times*, November 17, 1982

36. Dallman, M. et al. "Chronic stress and comfort foods: self-medication and abdominal obesity." *Brain, Behavior, and Immunity*. 2005, 19, 275–280.

37. Born JM, Lemmens SG, Rutters F, Nieuwenhuizen AG, Formisano E, Goebel R, Westerterp-Plantenga MS. "Acute stress and food-related reward activation in the brain during food choice during eating in the absence of hunger." *International Journal of Obesity*. 2010 Jan;34(1):172-81.

38. Wardle J, Cooke L. "The impact of obesity on psychological well-being." *Best Practice & Research Clinical Endocrinology*. 2005;19(3):421–40.

Chapter 5

39. *International Health Racquet and Sportsclub Association* Report 2012.

40. De Salles BF, Simão R, Fleck SJ, Dias I, Kraemer-Aguiar LG, Bouskela E. "Effects of resistance training on cytokines." *International Journal of Sports Medicine*. July 2010. 31 (7): 441–450.

41. Pedersen LR, Olsen RH, Jürs A, Astrup A, Chabanova E, Simonsen L, Wisløff U, Haugaard SB, Prescott E. "A randomised trial comparing weight loss with aerobic exercise in overweight individuals with coronary artery disease: The CUT-IT trial." *European Journal of Preventive Cardiology*. 2014 Jul 31.

42. Grego F1, Vallier JM, Collardeau M, Bermon S, Ferrari P, Candito M, Bayer P, Magnié MN, Brisswalter J. "Effects of long duration exercise on cognitive function, blood glucose, and counterregulatory hormones in male cyclists." *Neuroscience Letters*. 2004 Jul 1;364(2):76-80.

43. Hill EE, Zack E, Battaglini C, Viru M, Viru A, Hackney AC. "Exercise and circulating cortisol levels: the intensity threshold effect." *Journal of Endocrinological Investigation*. 2008 Jul;31(7):587-91.

Chapter 6

44. Manninen AH. "Is a calorie really a calorie? Metabolic advantage of low-carbohydrate diets." *Journal of the International Society of Sports Nutrition* 2004, 1(2):21-26.

45. Johnston CS, Day CS, Swan PD., *Postprandial thermogenesis is increased 100% on a high-protein, low-fat diet versus a high-carbohydrate, low-fat diet in healthy, young women.*, J Am Coll Nutr. 2002 Feb;21(1):55-61.

46. Vander Wal JS1, Marth JM, Khosla P, Jen KL, Dhurandhar NV. "Short-term effect of eggs on satiety in overweight and obese subjects." *Journal of the American College of Nutrition*. 2005 Dec; 24(6):510-5.

47. Wang S, Yang L, Lu J, Mu Y. "High-Protein Breakfast Promotes Weight Loss by Suppressing Subsequent Food Intake and Regulating Appetite Hormones in Obese Chinese Adolescents." *Hormone Research in Pediatrics*. 2014 Jun 11.

48. Liz Vaccariello "Flat Belly Diet" *Rodale* 2008,

49. Joaquín Pérez-Guisado, Andrés Muñoz-Serrano and Ángeles Alonso-Moraga. "Spanish Ketogenic Mediterranean diet: a healthy cardiovascular diet for weight loss.", *Nutrition Journal*. 2008; 7: 30.

50. Paniagua JA, Gallego de la Sacristana A, Romero I, Vidal-Puig A, Latre JM, Sanchez E, Perez-Martinez P, Lopez-Miranda J, Perez-Jimenez F. "Monounsaturated fat-rich diet prevents central body fat distribution and decreases postprandial adiponectin expression induced by a carbohydrate-rich diet in insulin-resistant subjects.", *Diabetes Care*. 2007 Jul; 30(7):1717-23.

51. Assunção ML, Ferreira HS, dos Santos AF, Cabral CR Jr, Florêncio TM. "Effects of dietary coconut oil on the biochemical and anthropometric profiles of women presenting abdominal obesity." *Lipids*. 2009 Jul;44(7):593-601.

52. Han JR, Deng B, Sun J, Chen CG, Corkey BE, Kirkland JL, Ma J, Guo W. "Effects of dietary medium-chain triglyceride on weight loss and insulin sensitivity in a group of moderately overweight free-living type 2 diabetic Chinese subjects." *Metabolism*. 2007 Jul;56(7):985-91.

53. Martínez-Fernández L, Laiglesia LM, Huerta AE, Martínez JA, Moreno-Aliaga MJ. "Omega-3 fatty acids and adipose tissue function in obesity and metabolic syndrome." *Prostaglandins and Other Lipid Mediators*. 2015 Jul 26.

54. Hätönen KA, Virtamo J, Eriksson JG, Sinkko HK, Sundvall JE, Valsta LM., Protein and fat modify the glycaemic and insulinaemic responses to a mashed potato-based meal. *British Journal of Nutrition*. 2011 Jul;106(2):248-53.

55. Andoh A, Tsujikawa T, Fujiyama Y. "Role of dietary fiber and short-chain fatty acids in the colon." *Current Pharmaceutical Design*. 2003;9(4):347-58.

56. D'Argenio G, Mazzacca G. "Short-chain fatty acid in the human colon. Relation to inflammatory bowel diseases and colon cancer." *Advances in Experimental Medicine and Biology*. 1999; 472:149-58.

57. Andoh A, Tsujikawa T, Fujiyama Y. "Role of dietary fiber and short-chain fatty acids in the colon." *Current Pharmaceutical Design*. 2003;9(4):347-58.

58. Rendo-Urteaga T, Puchau B, Chueca M, Oyarzabal M, Azcona-Sanjulián MC, Martínez JA, Marti A. "Total antioxidant capacity and oxidative stress after a 10-week dietary intervention program in obese children." *European Journal of Pediatrics*. 2013 Dec 6.

59. Puchau B, Zulet MA, de Echávarri AG, Hermsdorff HH, Martínez JA., "Dietary total antioxidant capacity is negatively associated with some metabolic syndrome features in healthy young adults." *Nutrition*. 2010 May;26(5):534-41.

60. Zulet MA, Puchau B, Hermsdorff HH, Navarro C, Martínez JA. "Vitamin A intake is inversely related with adiposity in healthy young adults." *Journal of Nutritional Science and Vitaminology* (Tokyo). 2008 Oct;54(5):347-52.

61. Folchetti LD, Monfort-Pires M, de Barros CR, Martini LA, Ferreira SR. "Association of fruits and vegetables consumption and related-vitamins with inflammatory and oxidative stress markers in prediabetic individuals." *Diabetololgy and Metabolic Syndrome*. 2014 Feb 18;6(1):22.

62. Pereira MA, Jacobs DR Jr., Van Horn L, Slattery ML, Kartashov AI, Ludwig DS., "Dairy consumption, obesity, and the insulin resistance syndrome in young adults: the CARDIA Study." *Journal of the American Medical Association*. 2002 Apr 24;287(16):2081-9.

63. Lee HJ, Cho JI, Lee HS, Kim CI, Cho E. "Intakes of dairy products and calcium and obesity in Korean adults: Korean National Health and Nutrition Examination Surveys (KNHANES) 2007-2009". *Public Library of Science*. 2014 Jun 10;9(6).

64. Johnson R, Bryant S, Huntley AL. "Green tea and green tea catechin extracts: An overview of the clinical evidence." *Maturitas*. 2012 Sep 14. pii: S0378-5122(12)00270-8.

65. Kim A, Chiu A, Barone MK, Avino D, Wang F, Coleman CI, Phung OJ. "Green tea catechins decrease total and low-density lipoprotein cholesterol: a systematic review and meta-analysis." *Journal of the American Dietetic Association*. 2011 Nov; 111(11):1720-9.

66. Westerterp-Plantenga MS, Lejeune MP, Kovacs EM. "Body weight loss and weight maintenance in relation to habitual caffeine intake and green tea supplementation." *Obesity research* 2005 Jul; 13(7):1195-204.

67. Thielecke F, Boschmann M. "The potential role of green tea catechins in the prevention of the metabolic syndrome - a review." *Phytochemistry*. 2009 Jan;70(1):11-24. Epub 2009 Jan 13.

Chapter 8

68. Jenkins DJH, Wolever TM, Taylor RH, et al. "Glycemic index of foods: a physiological basis for carbohydrate exchange." *The American Journal of Clinical Nutrition* 1981 Mar;34(3):362–6.

69. Sharon P.G. Fowler, Ken Williams and Helen P. Hazuda. "Diet Soda Intake Is Associated with Long-Term Increases in Waist Circumference in a Biethnic Cohort of Older Adults: The San Antonio Longitudinal Study of Aging (SALSA)." *Journal of the American Geriatrics Society* Volume 63, Issue 4, pages 708–715, April 2015.

70. Striegel Moore RH, Thompson D, Affenito SG, Franko DL, Obarzanek E, Barton BA, Schreiber GB, Daniels SR, Schmidt M, Crawford PB. "Correlates of beverage intake in adolescent girls: the National Heart, Lung, and Blood Institute Growth and Health Study." *Journal of Pediatrics*. 2006 Feb;148(2):183-7.

Appendix D

71. FDA Expands Advice on Statin Risks: http://www.fda.gov/ForConsumers/ConsumerUpdates/ucm293330.htm.

72. http://www.fda.gov/newsevents/newsroom/pressannouncements/ucm373939.htm.

73. Innis SM. "Dietary (omega-3) fatty acids and brain development. Nutrition Research Program, Child and Family Research Institute," *University of British Columbia*, Vancouver, BC V5Z 4H4, Canada.

74. Wainwright PE. "Dietary essential fatty acids and brain function: a developmental perspective on mechanisms." *Department of Health Studies and Gerontology*, University of Waterloo, Ontario, Canada.

75. Patterson E., Wall R.,Fitzgerald G. F., Ross R. P., Stanton C. "Health Implications of High Dietary Omega-6 Polyunsaturated Fatty Acids." *Journal of Nutrition and Metabolism* Volume 2012.

76. Simopoulos AP. "The importance of the ratio of omega-6/omega-3 essential fatty acids." *The Center for Genetics*, Nutrition and Health, Washington, DC 20009, USA.

77. "Evolutionary aspects of diet, the omega-6/omega-3 ratio and genetic variation: nutritional implications for chronic diseases."*The Center for Genetics, Nutrition and Health*, Washington, DC 20009, USA.

78. Simopoulos AP. "The importance of the ratio of omega-6/omega-3 essential fatty acids." *The Center for Genetics*, Nutrition and Health.

79. Rees AM, Austin MP, Parker G (April 2005). "Role of omega-3 fatty acids as a treatment for depression in the perinatal period". *The Australian and New Zealand Journal of Psychiatry* 39 (4): 274–80.

80. A. Jenkinson, A. R. Collins, S. J. Duthie, K. W. J. Wahle and G. G. Duthie. "The effect of increased intakes of polyunsaturated fatty acids and vitamin E on DNA damage in human lymphocytes." *The Federation of American Societies for Experimental Biology Journal*, vol. 13 no. 15 2138-2142.

81. Brenna JT. "Efficiency of conversion of alpha-linolenic acid to long chain n-3 fatty acids in man." *Current Opinion in Clinical Nutrition & Metabolic Care*. 2002 Mar;5(2):127-32.

82. "Fats and fatty acids in human nutrition, Report of an expert consultation." *Food and Agriculture Organisation Food and Nutrition*, 10 – 14 November 2008, Geneva.

83. Lands, William E.M. "Dietary fat and health: the evidence and the politics of prevention: careful use of dietary fats can improve life and prevent disease." *Annals of the New York* Academy of Sciences (Blackwell), December 2005, 1055: 179–192.

84. Hibbeln, Joseph R., Nieminen, Levi R.G., Blasbalg, Tanya L., Riggs, Jessica A., Lands, William E. M., (1). "Healthy intakes of n–3 and n–6 fatty acids: estimations considering worldwide diversity." *American Journal of Clinical Nutrition*, June 2006, 83: 1483S–1493S.

85. Sonestedt, Emily; Ericson, Ulrika; Gullberg, Bo; Skog, Kerstin; Olsson, Håkan; Wirfält, Elisabet (2008). "Do both heterocyclic amines and omega-6 polyunsaturated fatty acids contribute to the incidence of breast cancer in postmenopausal women of the Malmö diet and cancer cohort?" *The International Journal of Cancer* (International Union Against Cancer) 123 (7): 1637–1643.

86. Yong Q. Chen, at al (2007). "Modulation of prostate cancer genetic risk by omega-3 and omega-6 fatty acids." *The Journal of Clinical Investigation* 117 (7): 1866–1875.

Appendix E

87. Keys A, Taylor HL, Blackburn H, Brozek J, Anderson JT, Simonson E., "Coronary Heart Disease among Minnesota Business and Professional Men Followed Fifteen Years.", *Circulation* 28:381-95 (Sept 1963).

88. Siri-Tarino PW, Sun Q, Hu FB, Krauss RM. "Meta-analysis of prospective cohort studies evaluating the association of saturated fat with cardiovascular disease." *American Journal of Clinical Nutrition*. 2010;91:535-46.

89. Micha R, Mozaffarian D. "Saturated fat and cardiometabolic risk factors, coronary heart disease, stroke, and diabetes: a fresh look at the evidence." *Lipids*. 2010;45:893-905.

90. Rizzo M., Berneis K.. "Low-density lipoprotein size and cardiovascular risk assessment." *Quarterly Journal of Medicine*, January 2006 99 (1): 1-14.

91. Packard CJ. "Small dense low-density lipoprotein and its role as an independent predictor of cardiovascular disease." *Current Opinion in Lipidology*. 2006 Aug;17(4):412-7.

92. Steinberg, D. "Low density lipoprotein oxidation and its pathobiological significance." *Journal of Biological Chemistry*, 1997, 272.

93. Griffin, B. A., Freeman, D. J., Tait, G. W., Thomson, J., Caslake, M. J., Packard, C. J. & Shepherd, J. "Role of plasma triglyceride in the regulation of plasma low density lipoprotein (LDL) subfractions: relative contribution of small, dense LDL to coronary heart disease risk." *Atherosclerosis*, 1994, 106:241-253.

94. Kazumasa Yamagishi, Hiroyasu Iso, Hiroshi Yatsuya, Naohito Tanabe, Chigusa Date, Shogo Kikuchi, Akio Yamamoto, Yutaka Inaba, and Akiko Tamakoshi. "Dietary intake of saturated fatty acids and mortality from cardiovascular disease in Japanese: the Japan Collaborative Cohort Study for Evaluation of Cancer Risk (JACC) Study." *American Journal of Clinical Nutrition*. October 2010 vol. 92 no. 4 759-765.

95. Gillman MW, Cupples LA, Millen BE, Ellison RC, Wolf PA. "Inverse association of dietary fat with development of ischemic stroke in men." *Journal of the American Medical Association* 1997;278:2145–50.

96. He K., Merchant A., Rimm EB, Rosner BA, Stampfer MJ, Willett WC, Ascherio A. "Dietary fat intake and risk of stroke in male US healthcare professionals: 14 year prospective cohort study." *British Medical Journal*, 2003 Oct 4;327(7418):777-82.

97. Dr. Aseem Malhotra. "Saturated fat is not the major issue." *British Medical Journal* 2013; 347.

98. Guay V., Lamarche B., Charest A., Tremblay AJ, Couture P. "Effect of short-term low- and high-fat diets on low-density lipoprotein particle size in normolipidemic subjects." *Metabolism*, 2012 Jan;61(1):76-83.

99. Sharman MJ, Kraemer WJ, Love DM, Avery NG, Gómez AL, Scheett TP, Volek JS. "A ketogenic diet favorably affects serum biomarkers for cardiovascular disease in normal-weight men." *Journal of Nutrition*, 2002 Jul;132(7):1879-85.

100. Parks, E. J. & Hellerstein, M. K. (2000) Carbohydrate-induced hypertriacylglycerolemia: historical perspective and review of biological mechanisms. *American Journal of Clinical Nutrition*. 71:412-433.

101. Assunção ML, Ferreira HS, dos Santos AF, Cabral CR Jr, Florêncio TM., Effects of dietary coconut oil on the biochemical and anthropometric profiles of women presenting abdominal obesity., *Lipids*. 2009 Jul;44(7):593-601.

102. Owen CG, Whincup PH, Cook DG., Breast-feeding and cardiovascular risk factors and outcomes in later life: evidence from epidemiological studies., *Proceedings of the Nutrition Society*. 2011 Nov;70(4):478-84.

103. Fewtrell MS., Breast-feeding and later risk of CVD and obesity: evidence from randomised trials., *Proceedings of the Nutrition Society*. 2011 Nov;70(4):472-7.

104. Christopher D. Gardner, PhD; Alexandre Kiazand, MD; Sofiya Alhassan, PhD; Soowon Kim, PhD; Randall S. Stafford, MD, PhD; Raymond R. Balise, PhD; Helena C. Kraemer, PhD; Abby C. King, PhD., Comparison of the Atkins, Zone, Ornish, and LEARN Diets for Change in Weight and Related Risk Factors Among Overweight Premenopausal Women: The A TO Z Weight Loss Study: A Randomized Trial., *Journal of the American Medical Association*. 2007;297(9):969-977.

105. Jean Ferrières., The French paradox: lessons for other countries. *Heart*. 2004 January; 90(1): 107–111.

106. S L Malhotra., Epidemiology of ischaemic heart disease in India with special reference to causation., *British Heart Journal*. 1967 November; 29(6): 895–905.

107. http://www.fda.gov/forconsumers/consumerupdates/ucm293330.htm.

108. Maciej Gasior, Michael A. Rogawski, and Adam L. Hartman, Neuroprotective and disease-modifying effects of the ketogenic diet, *Behavioural Pharmacology*. 2006 September; 17(5-6): 431–439.

109. Murphy P., Likhodii S., Nylen K., Burnham WM., The antidepressant properties of the ketogenic diet. *Biological Psychiatry*. 2004 Dec 15;56(12):981-3.

110. http://www.lpch.org/clinicalSpecialtiesServices/ClinicalSpecialties/Neurology/neurology.html

111. Aneja A., Tierney E., Autism: The Role of Cholesterol in Treatment. *International Review of Psychiatry*, 2008 Apr 20(2):165-70).

112. http://archives.cnn.com/2000/HEALTH/men/06/30/low.cholesterol.wmd/index.html.

113. Texas A&M University (2008, January 10). Surprise — Cholesterol May Actually Pose Benefits. *Science Daily*.

114. WHO cooperative trial on primary prevention of ischemic heart disease with clofibrate to lower serum cholesterol: final mortality follow-up. Report of the Committee of Principal Investigators. *Lancet* 1984; 2:600-4.

115. Scott R, Best J, Forder P, Taskinen MR, Simes J, Barter P, Keech A. Fenofibrate Intervention and Event Lowering in Diabetes (FIELD) study: baseline characteristics and short-term effects of fenofibrate. *Cardiovascular Diabetology* 2005 Aug 22;4:13.

116. Kritchevsky SB., Kritchevsky D., Serum cholesterol and cancer risk: an epidemiologic perspective. *Annual Review of Nutrition*. 1992;12:391-416.

117. Ravnskov U., McCully K. S., and Rosch P.J., The statin-low cholesterol-cancer conundrum., Quarterly *Journal of Medicine* (Association of Physicians). 2012 Apr;105(4):383-8.

118. American College of Cardiology. "Low LDL cholesterol is related to cancer risk.", *Science Daily*, 26 March 2012.

119. Benn M, Tybjærg-Hansen A, Stender S, Frikke-Schmidt R, Nordestgaard BG., "Low-density lipoprotein cholesterol and the risk of cancer: a mendelian randomization study." *Journal of the National Cancer Institute* 2011 Mar 16;103(6):508-19.

Appendix F

120. Cerami A., "Hypothesis. Glucose as a mediator of aging." *Journal of the American Geriatrics Society*. Soc. 33:626–634. 1985.

121. Kenneth B. Beckman , Bruce N. Ames., "The Free Radical Theory of Aging Matures.", *Physiological Reviews*, Vol. 78 no. 547-581, 1 April 1998.

122. Thornalley PJ., "Advanced glycation end products in renal failure." *Journal of Renal Nutrition*. 2006 Jul;16(3):178-84.

123. Ahmed N., "Advanced glycation endproducts--role in pathology of diabetic complications." *Diabetes Research and Clinical Practice*. 2005 Jan;67(1):3-21.

124. Soldatos, G., Cooper ME. "Advanced glycation end products and vascular structure and function." *Current Hypertension Reports* 8 (6): 472–478. Dec 2006.

125. Baynes JW, Thorpe SR. "Glycoxidation and lipoxidation in atherogenesis." *Free Radical Biology & Medicine* 28: 1708-1716, 2000.

126. Ohnuki Y, Nagano R, Takizawa S, Takagi S, Miyata T., "Advanced glycation end products in patients with cerebral infarction." *Internal Medicine*. 2009;48(8):587-91.

127. Tousoulis D, Zisimos K, Antoniades C, et al. "Oxidative stress and inflammatory process in patients with atrial fibrillation: the role of left atrium distension." *International Journal of Cardiology*. 2008.

128. Ishibashi T, Murata T, Hangai M, Nagai R, Horiuchi S, Lopez PF, Hinton DR, Ryan SJ., "Advanced glycation end products in age-related macular degeneration." *Archives of ophthalmology*. 1998 Dec;116(12):1629-32.

129. Koschinsky T, He CJ, Mitsuhashi T, et al., "Orally absorbed reactive glycation products (glycotoxins): an environmental risk factor in diabetic nephropathy". *Proceedings of the National Academy of Sciences* U.S.A. 94 (12): 6474–9.June 1997.

130. Levi B and Werman M., "Long-Term Fructose Consumption Accelerates Glycation and Several Age-Related Variables in Male Rats." *Journal of Nutrition*September 1, 1998 vol. 128 no. 9 1442-1449.

131. Shapiro A1, Mu W, Roncal C, Cheng KY, Johnson RJ, Scarpace PJ. "Fructose-induced leptin resistance exacerbates weight gain in response to subsequent high-fat feeding.", *American journal of physiology*. Regulatory, integrative and comparative physiology. 2008 Nov;295(5).

Appendix G

132. Bamm VV, Tsemakhovich VA, Shaklai N. "Oxidation of low-density lipoprotein by hemoglobin–hemichrome." *The International Journal of Biochemistry & Cell Biology*. 2003;35(3):349-58.

133. http://www.nhlbi.nih.gov/health/health-topics/topics/heartattack.

134. http://www.nhlbi.nih.gov/health/health-topics/topics/stroke/types.

135. Butterfield DA, Castegna A, Lauderback CM, Drake J., "Evidence that amyloid beta-peptide-induced lipid peroxidation and its sequelae in Alzheimer's disease brain contribute to neuronal death." *Neurobiology of Aging*. 2002 Sep-Oct; 23(5):655-64.

136. Floyd RA, Carney JM., "Free radical damage to protein and DNA: mechanisms involved and relevant observations on brain undergoing oxidative stress." *Annals of Neurology* 1992; 32 Suppl:S22-7.

137. Takahashi S, Takahashi I, Sato H, Kubota Y, Yoshida S, Muramatsu Y., "Age-related changes in the concentrations of major and trace elements in the brain of rats and mice." *Biological Trace Element Research*. 2001 May; 80(2):145-58.

138. Atwood CS, Obrenovich ME, Liu T, Chan H, Perry G, Smith MA, Martins RN., "Amyloid-beta: a chameleon walking in two worlds: a review of the trophic and toxic properties of amyloid-beta." *Brain Research Reviews*. 2003 Sep; 43(1):1-16.

139. Lotharius J, Brundin P., "Impaired dopamine storage resulting from alpha-synuclein mutations may contribute to the pathogenesis of Parkinson's disease." *Human Molecular Genetics*. 2002 Oct 1; 11(20):2395-407.

140. Cadet JL. "Free radical mechanisms in the central nervous system: An overview." *International Journal of Neuroscience*. 1998;40:13–18.

141. Demopoulos HB, Flamm ES, Pietronigro DD, Seligman ML., "The free radical pathology and the microcirculation in the major central nervous system disorders." *Acta physiologica Scandinavica. Supplementum*. 1980; 492:91-119.

142. Yoshikawa T., "Free radicals and their scavengers in Parkinson's disease." *European Neurology*. 1993; 33 Suppl 1:60-8.

143. Dizdaroglu M, Jaruga P. "Mechanisms of free radical-induced damage to DNA." *Free Radical Research*. 2012;46(4):382-419.

144. Pageon H, Asselineau D. "An in Vitro Approach to the Chronological Aging of Skin by Glycation of the Collagen: The Biological Effect of Glycation on the Reconstructed Skin Model." *Annals of the New York Academy of Sciences*. 2005;1043(1):529-32.

145. Palermo V, Mattivi F, Silvestri R, La Regina G, Falcone C, Mazzoni C., "Apple can act as anti-aging on yeast cells.", *Current Pharmaceutical Design*. Aug 2012;2012:491759.

146. Aviram M., Dornfeld L., Rosenblat M. "Pomegranate juice consumption reduces oxidative stress, atherogenic modification to LDL, and platelet aggregation: studies in humans and in atherosclerotic apolipoprotein E-deficient mice." *American Journal of Clinical Nutrition*. 2000; 71: 1062-1076.

147. Aviram M., Rosenblat M., Gaitini D. "Pomegranate juice consumption for 3 years by patients with carotid artery stenosis reduces common carotid intima-media thickness, blood pressure and LDL oxidation." *Clinical Nutrition*. 2004; 23: 423-433.

148. Brambilla D., Mancuso C., Scuderi M.R., Bosco P., Cantarella G., Lempereur L., et al. «The role of antioxidant supplement in immune system, neoplastic, and neurodegenerative disorders: a point of view for an assessment of the risk/benefit profile.", *Nutrition Journal* 2008; 7: 29-35.

149. Bonnefoy M, Drai J, Kostka T. "Antioxidants to slow aging, facts and perspectives.", *Presse Med*. 2002 Jul 27;31(25):1174-84.

150. Gerhauser C., "Cancer chemopreventive potential of apples, apple juice, and apple components.", *Planta Medica*. 2008 Oct;74(13):1608-24. Epub 2008 Oct 14.

151. Lin YT, Wang LF, Hsu YC., "Curcuminoids suppress the growth of pharynx and nasopharyngeal carcinoma cells through induced apoptosis.", *Journal of Agricultural and Food Chemistry*. 2009 May 13;57(9):3765-70.

152. Chang CC, Fu CF, Yang WT, Chen TY, Hsu YC., "The cellular uptake and cytotoxic effect of curcuminoids on breast cancer cells.", *Taiwan Journal of Obstetrics and Gynaecology*. 2012 Sep;51(3):368-74.

153. Hsu YC, Weng HC, Lin S, Chien YW., "Curcuminoids-cellular uptake by human primary colon cancer cells as quantitated by a sensitive HPLC assay and its relation with the inhibition of proliferation and apoptosis.", *Journal of Agricultural and Food Chemistry*. 2007 Oct 3;55(20):8213-22.

154. Lopresti AL, Hood SD, Drummond PD. "Multiple antidepressant potential modes of action of curcumin: a review of its anti-inflammatory, monoaminergic, antioxidant, immune-modulating and neuroprotective effects.", *Journal of Psychopharmacology*. 2012 Oct 3.

155. Kulkarni S, Dhir A, Akula KK.. "Potentials of curcumin as an antidepressant.", *Scientific World Journal*. 2009 Nov 1;9:1233-41.

156. Mythri RB, Bharath MM. "Curcumin: a potential neuroprotective agent in Parkinson's disease.", *Current Pharmaceutical Design*. 2012; 18(1):91-9.

Coming Soon:
Skinny Without Willpower Cookbook

Daily Food Diary

Diary for __/__/20__

BREAKFAST

Food Group **Food Item and Amount**

Vegetables

Fruits

Dairy

Grains/Lentils

Protein

Fat

Nuts

Herbs/Spices

Comments

MID-MORNING SNACK

Food Group **Food Item and Amount**

LUNCH

Food Group	Food Item and Amount
Vegetables	
Fruits	
Dairy	
Grains/Lentils	
Protein	
Fat	
Nuts	
Herbs/Spices	
Comments	

MID-AFTERNOON SNACK

Food Group	Food Item and Amount

DINNER

Food Group	Food Item and Amount
Vegetables	
Fruits	
Dairy	
Grains/Lentils	
Protein	
Fat	
Nuts	
Herbs/Spices	
Comments	

BEDTIME SNACK

Food Group	Food Item and Amount

Diary for ___/___/20___

BREAKFAST

Food Group	Food Item and Amount
Vegetables	
Fruits	
Dairy	
Grains/Lentils	
Protein	
Fat	
Nuts	
Herbs/Spices	
Comments	

MID-MORNING SNACK

Food Group	Food Item and Amount

LUNCH

Food Group	Food Item and Amount
Vegetables	
Fruits	
Dairy	
Grains/Lentils	
Protein	
Fat	
Nuts	
Herbs/Spices	
Comments	

MID-AFTERNOON SNACK

Food Group	Food Item and Amount

DINNER

Food Group	Food Item and Amount
Vegetables	
Fruits	
Dairy	
Grains/Lentils	
Protein	
Fat	
Nuts	
Herbs/Spices	
Comments	

BEDTIME SNACK

Food Group	Food Item and Amount

Diary for __/__/20__

BREAKFAST

Food Group	Food Item and Amount
Vegetables	
Fruits	
Dairy	
Grains/Lentils	
Protein	
Fat	
Nuts	
Herbs/Spices	
Comments	

MID-MORNING SNACK

Food Group	Food Item and Amount

LUNCH

Food Group	Food Item and Amount
Vegetables	
Fruits	
Dairy	
Grains/Lentils	
Protein	
Fat	
Nuts	
Herbs/Spices	
Comments	

MID-AFTERNOON SNACK

Food Group	Food Item and Amount

DINNER

Food Group	Food Item and Amount
Vegetables	
Fruits	
Dairy	
Grains/Lentils	
Protein	
Fat	
Nuts	
Herbs/Spices	
Comments	

BEDTIME SNACK

Food Group	Food Item and Amount

Diary for __/__/20__

BREAKFAST

Food Group **Food Item and Amount**

Vegetables

Fruits

Dairy

Grains/Lentils

Protein

Fat

Nuts

Herbs/Spices

Comments

MID-MORNING SNACK

Food Group **Food Item and Amount**

LUNCH

Food Group	Food Item and Amount
Vegetables	
Fruits	
Dairy	
Grains/Lentils	
Protein	
Fat	
Nuts	
Herbs/Spices	
Comments	

MID-AFTERNOON SNACK

Food Group	Food Item and Amount

DINNER

Food Group	Food Item and Amount
Vegetables	
Fruits	
Dairy	
Grains/Lentils	
Protein	
Fat	
Nuts	
Herbs/Spices	
Comments	

BEDTIME SNACK

Food Group	Food Item and Amount

Diary for ___/___/20___

BREAKFAST

Food Group	Food Item and Amount
Vegetables	
Fruits	
Dairy	
Grains/Lentils	
Protein	
Fat	
Nuts	
Herbs/Spices	
Comments	

MID-MORNING SNACK

Food Group	Food Item and Amount

LUNCH

Food Group	Food Item and Amount
Vegetables	
Fruits	
Dairy	
Grains/Lentils	
Protein	
Fat	
Nuts	
Herbs/Spices	
Comments	

MID-AFTERNOON SNACK

Food Group	Food Item and Amount

DINNER

Food Group	Food Item and Amount
Vegetables	
Fruits	
Dairy	
Grains/Lentils	
Protein	
Fat	
Nuts	
Herbs/Spices	
Comments	

BEDTIME SNACK

Food Group	Food Item and Amount

Diary for ___/___/20___

BREAKFAST

Food Group	Food Item and Amount
Vegetables	
Fruits	
Dairy	
Grains/Lentils	
Protein	
Fat	
Nuts	
Herbs/Spices	
Comments	

MID-MORNING SNACK

Food Group	Food Item and Amount

LUNCH

Food Group	Food Item and Amount
Vegetables	
Fruits	
Dairy	
Grains/Lentils	
Protein	
Fat	
Nuts	
Herbs/Spices	
Comments	

MID-AFTERNOON SNACK

Food Group	Food Item and Amount

DINNER

Food Group	Food Item and Amount
Vegetables	
Fruits	
Dairy	
Grains/Lentils	
Protein	
Fat	
Nuts	
Herbs/Spices	
Comments	

BEDTIME SNACK

Food Group	Food Item and Amount

Diary for ___/___/20___

BREAKFAST

Food Group	Food Item and Amount
Vegetables	
Fruits	
Dairy	
Grains/Lentils	
Protein	
Fat	
Nuts	
Herbs/Spices	
Comments	

MID-MORNING SNACK

Food Group	Food Item and Amount

LUNCH

Food Group	Food Item and Amount
Vegetables	
Fruits	
Dairy	
Grains/Lentils	
Protein	
Fat	
Nuts	
Herbs/Spices	
Comments	

MID-AFTERNOON SNACK

Food Group	Food Item and Amount

DINNER

Food Group	Food Item and Amount
Vegetables	
Fruits	
Dairy	
Grains/Lentils	
Protein	
Fat	
Nuts	
Herbs/Spices	
Comments	

BEDTIME SNACK

Food Group	Food Item and Amount

CPSIA information can be obtained at www.ICGtesting.com
Printed in the USA
LVOW08s1359280416

485760LV00004B/165/P